# The Gift of Ruth

## Love is a gift bestowed from heaven

### By Jay Carp

*River Pointe Publications • Milan, Michigan, USA*

# The Gift of Ruth

First American Paperback edition
Large Print

River Pointe Publications
P.O. Box 234, Milan, MI 48160, USA

Library of Congress Cataloging-in-Publication Data

Carp, Jay.
 The gift of Ruth : love is a gift bestowed from Heaven / by Jay Carp.
-- 1st American pbk. ed.
     p. cm.
ISBN 978-0-9758805-9-3 (lg. print : pbk. : alk.paper)
1. Carp, Jay. 2. Carp, Ruth Ormondroyd. 3. Cancer--Patients--Mich-igan--Biography. 4. Electronics engineers--Michigan--Biography. 5. Man-woman relationships--Michigan. 6. Love--Michigan. 7. Michi-gan--Biography. 8. Massachusetts--Biography.
l. Title.
CT275.C3133A3 2008
362.196'9949092--dc22
                    2008015950

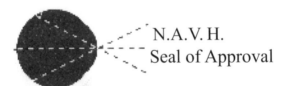

N.A.V.H.
Seal of Approval

Cover design by Barbara J. Gunia, Sans Serif, Inc.
Cover photograph: Ruth Ormondroyd

*Printed in U.S.A.*

*Jay Carp*

# Contents

# The Gift of Ruth

# LIFE IS A JOURNEY ENRICHED BY AGE

The young attach little significance to the significant fact that they are alive; it is only as we grow older that we begin to appreciate and treasure what we have. Youngsters chugalug their experiences because they believe that their future is endless; oldsters savor their experiences because they know that their future has limits. Maturity requires time but its reward is to give us a sense of what is meaningful. Age takes away the feeling of immortality, but in exchange, age bestows a degree of wisdom.

As a young man I was as oblivious to the meaning of life as I was aware of the facts of life. And that of course is normal. When you are young and your future is limitless why ponder what might happen tomorrow? No young person ever plans to age.

Like most young people, I associated almost entirely with people of my own age and I paid scant attention to older people. They were around, and, except for an occasional teacher or two, they didn't intrude upon my world. Of course I loved my parents and grandparents but I thought of them simply as role models along my path. They were like roadside billboards, large, two-dimensional, and with big messages.

When I was young it never occurred to me that older people could be filled with the same passions and emotions that I was experiencing. Except for an occasional outburst, older people appeared to be settled and subdued and I assumed that they had weathered all the traumas of their lives and that their age had given them serenity.

Life has taught me that my youthful assumption was completely wrong. Happiness has no warranty and it can be snatched away without notice. I know because I am now sixty-nine years old and my life has just been crushed, like a teacup under a truck tire, by the death of my beloved wife. The loss of her wit, her charm, her beauty, her humanity, totally haunts me. I ache for her, but to no avail. She is gone.

But her memories remain and they constantly torment me. Not a day passes without a reminder of Ruth. It could be the refrain of a song on the radio, or a contrail slowly making its way across the blue sky, or a piece of junk mail with her name on it. I have no understanding of, and no control over, these memories and how they start. They just appear and overwhelm me wherever I am. As a result, I find myself weeping in the oddest places, at the oddest times, over the oddest things. My grief shows me no mercy.

I want things to go back to the way they were before Ruth's death and, of course, they never will. Love is sweet when you have a partner, love is bitter when you are alone. My love for my wife did not stop at her death, and the pain of my loss has left me hollow and lonely.

Ruth would not want me dwelling on these thoughts, as she was never one to wallow in self-pity. Even after she discovered that her cancer was spreading and that she was going to die, she insisted on carrying on with the business of life. First, she talked with me and told me what she wanted and needed from me. Then, she called her daughters and told them what she expected of them. If she could be that strong, then I must also be that strong. I would always want her to be proud of me.

Whenever Ruth had the opportunity to talk about us, she would say, "Jay and I were engaged to each other in 1950, but, we were not married until 1993." Although she would make the re-mark casually, she would be carefully watch-ing for the reaction. Invariably, the subject being discussed would come to a standstill and the person she was talking to would ask for a more complete explanation.

Actually, I was the one that began telling people about us after we first got married. I was so proud and so happy to be her husband that I wanted everyone to know our story.

And at first Ruth didn't like me saying anything as she was a very private person. But, after she thought about it, and as her happiness overcame her reticence, she began to change her mind. Our marriage amazed her as much as it did me and she enjoyed describing how we first met, how we broke up, and how we eventually came back together again.

It really didn't matter which one of us began to tell our story because some of the events had taken place so long ago that we each had to buttress the other's memory. She would ask me to remember the name of a mutual acquaintance or I would ask her to recall the details of some past event. There were things that I had forgotten, there were things that Ruth had forgotten, and there were memories that neither of us would ever forget.

There is nothing I can do that will bring Ruth back to me and I cannot stop my pain. However, I can do what Ruth delighted in doing. I can tell our story. Even though our love made us husband and wife late in our lives, I find myself dividing our time together in parallel with the seasons of the year. Spring was our awakening, summer was our sweetness, fall was our harvest, and winter was our death.

## SPRING

The first time I saw Ruth was at a bus stop on Wallingford Street in Ann Arbor. It was the fall of 1948 and I was starting my junior year at the University of Michigan. The fraternity I had joined at the end of my sophomore year had just moved into a new house on Hermitage Road, which ran into Wallingford a few hundred feet from our front door. The new house was further away from the campus than the previous location but it was bigger and housed more members. The easiest way to get to the university from the edge of the city and avoid the terrible parking problems around the campus was to take the bus.

I had overslept and I had to hurry to get to my first morning class of the new semester. The bus came into view as I started out the front door and, so as not to miss it, I began to trot towards the bus stop. As I got close, I saw four or five of my fraternity brothers gathered around a tall blond girl and talking with her. I did not see her face because her back was to me. When the bus stopped, everyone got on in the front and made their way down through the bus looking for empty seats. Just as it started to pull away I dashed through the rear door and stood in the back holding on to a pole.

I looked towards the front of the bus and saw the girl who had been talking with my fraternity brothers. I watched her walk past two or three rows of seats before sitting down and I think my heart must have stopped beating for an instant. If God had opened the door and invited me into Heaven, I couldn't have been more awed. Ruth was the most beautiful girl I had ever seen. She was tall, over five foot ten inches, and she carried herself gracefully. She had long blond hair, green eyes and a face that could make the angels sing. I stared and stared and, when she sat down, I kept my eyes fixed on the back of her head. My heart filled with joy, and my eyes almost welled. I was glad to be in the back by myself because I didn't want anyone noticing my reaction. I don't even remember getting off the bus.

For the next few weeks I got to the bus stop early every day just so I could watch Ruth walk from her house to the bus stop. When she arrived, my fraternity brothers would immediately surround her and vie for her attention.

She obviously enjoyed having an audience and she talked with everyone without singling out anyone for special attention. She was totally engaged with her entourage.

I was the only exception. Bewitched by her beauty, I could not muster the courage to join the group and enter the conversation. I was helpless to do anything but stare at her and worship her from a distance. When she got off the bus, I would follow her across campus watching her move as she walked. If her hair was held back in a ponytail, there would be a rhythm between the sway of her hips and the bobbing of her hair. It was a sweet, almost innocent, eroticism. Ruth fascinated me.

Although I felt fortunate every day just to be able to look at her, I could not bring myself to walk over and enter her circle of admirers and join in the conversation. Despite being at a distance and hearing only fragments of what was being said, I watched Ruth's face mirror her reactions. She would smile, or be serious, or frown, or once or twice, show disgust at an off color remark.

My problem was that my wildest dream and my worst nightmare were both being answered at the same time. Because I had always been timid around girls, I was lonely. I yearned for a girl friend, someone with whom I could share life's adventures. In the past, I had met and dated several girls but I had not established any romantic attachments. The spark that ignites and welds that bond had never been struck. Meeting this gorgeous, vital woman would have been the answer to all of my dreams.

And that is where my nightmare kicked in. My dream had not only been answered, it had been totally fulfilled, and I was afraid to try and take advantage of it. Ruth was so stunning that she took my breath away. She seemed so complete in looks, charm, and personality that I didn't have the courage to speak to her. I was sure that, by her standards, I would just be boring and dull. Although I possessed a sense of humor and was an easy conversationalist, I was fearful that my social skills were not enough to interest this golden goddess. I couldn't bear the thought of her laughing at me or rejecting me, so I avoided the group that surrounded her. Lack of self-confidence forced me to be an onlooker when I really wanted to be a participant.

But what I could do, and did do, was listen in on any conversation in the fraternity house whenever her name was mentioned. Every scrap of information was a bonbon. I learned that her name was Ruth Ormondroyd. She lived around the corner on Copley Road and she was a Liberal Arts student majoring in French. Her father was a Professor of Engineering at Michigan and she took the bus because her father refused to drive to campus despite his having a reserved parking place. No matter what the weather was like, he insisted on walking the two and a half miles to, and from, the School of Engineering every day.

I collected details on Ruth more avidly than a miser hoards gold pieces. I had never felt like this about anyone, and since I couldn't bring myself to talk to her, the best I could do was eavesdrop. To me, it seemed like time was measured only by our shared bus trips to campus. I must have shown up at classes, studied, taken exams, gone to the football games, and dated, but whatever I did, I found myself dreaming that I did it with Ruth.

Weeks went by, the weather started to take on a chill and soon the fall semester would be coming to an end. I began to be concerned that her class schedule for the next semester might not coincide with mine and that we wouldn't be taking the bus at the same time.

And then we bumped into each other. Literally.

Angell Hall is a large, impressive, structure with massive granite pillars and a wide staircase sweeping up to its front entrances. The first floor is filled with huge lecture halls, each seating several hundred students. One afternoon, I was making my way out of one of these rooms after a lecture. It was always difficult to thread a path through the mob of students because some are trying to get out quickly, some are trying to get in slowly, and some are just talking and not moving either way. I walked ahead impatiently and inadvertently I brushed against someone who came towards me from the side.

"Excuse me," I said, reacting without even seeing the person I had made contact with. Turning, I found myself looking directly into Ruth Ormondroyd's deep green eyes. That impersonal jostle, along with her sudden closeness, shocked me into speaking.

"You are Ruth."

She smiled and I felt my shell of silence melt away. She replied, "And you are Jay."

It turned out that we had both been taking this course almost all semester long. I usually sat up in front and had never noticed her in such a large class. Ruth sat in the back and she had not noticed me either. This particular day, She was hurrying to meet one of her girl friends at the door towards which we were both heading. We waited outside of the classroom for about ten minutes and when her friend didn't show up we left together. It wasn't until years after we were married that Ruth told me the entire truth about that meeting.

I can't recall any details about the rest of that day, and neither could Ruth. I know that we had coffee at the Women's League, and I know that we talked about everything and we talked about nothing. We finally caught the last bus back home. On that late fall day, the floodgates of my youthful love and happiness burst wide open.

The next morning I was at the bus stop, off to one side as usual, and I was apprehensive, not knowing what to expect from Ruth. I kept thinking that perhaps our time together had not been as important or as enjoyable to her as it had been to me. Or perhaps I had bored her or made her angry. Or perhaps she had been play-ing with me because she wanted a new mouse for her cat game. All I could do was hope for the best and expect the worst. The joy of yesterday seemed to taste bitter today.

Finally, Ruth came around the corner and walked over to where we were waiting for the bus. She paused briefly and talked for a while with my fraternity brothers and then she came over and stood beside me. As she did, I heard one of them say loudly, "Hey, what's going on here? When the hell did Jay get into the act?" I paid no attention–my eyes were on Ruth. We boarded the bus together, sat down beside each other, and from that moment on, Ruth became the axis around which my entire world rotated.

It seems as if the remainder of that year went by with incredible speed. We were awash in attraction for each other and we hardly ever stopped talking and laughing. We were together constantly, enjoying all the things that college life presented in Ann Arbor. We went to the Pretzel Bell and drank beer by the pitcher. We went to football games, hockey games, movies, attended concerts, dined out with her parents, and walked through the Arboretum. We would go canoeing up the Huron River, with a case of beer, and picnic with three or four other couples. I am almost sure that we even managed to get to our classes and take our exams.

I had never learned to dance, so the one thing we didn't often do was go dancing. Ruth enjoyed dancing and periodically she would suggest that we go to a fraternity dance or a prom. When we did, all I could do was shuffle my feet in time to the music. She did not volunteer to teach me and I am sure that was because I did not think of asking her. She understood that I was embarrassed and uncomfortable at my lack of dancing skills so she never discussed it.

All of our activities were done with mutual friends from a wide background. Some were our classmates but we also spent time with my fraternity brothers and some athletes from the football team. Ruth, having lived in Ann Arbor almost all of her life, had a large group of girl-friends from high school, some of them attend-ed Michigan, and many did not. It really didn't matter who was with us or what we did, as long as we were together. We just couldn't get enough of each other.

A marvelous thing had happened to me. I had met a woman who stirred my thoughts and feelings just by holding my hand. Being with her made me want to be a better person. For me, life had become mandolins and moonlight, blue-birds and blueberries.

I was in love.

Although I was swimming in a sea of hap-piness, I sometimes had fears of drowning. I couldn't believe that Ruth had chosen me. I con-sidered myself blessed, but deep inside of me, I felt uneasy. I occasionally wondered if Ruth would simply tire of me and want to break up.

From the time that we first met, it was ob-vious to both of us that we came from different backgrounds. That made no difference to Ruth, and, as a matter of fact, it may have even made me more attractive to her as she told me that she had never met anyone quite like me. Of course, we were both curious about each other's past.

My doubts about us began when I became

aware of the lifestyle of Ruth and her family. The Ormondroyds were a family that was well to do, orderly, educated and Protestant.

My family, in comparison, stood in sad contrast to the Ormondroyds. We were not well to do; we ran the gamut from poor to middle class. We were not orderly; we were completely disorganized. So much so, that I never invited any of my friends over to my house. They had clean, neat homes. Our kitchen table and our sink usually were stacked with dirty dishes. Our chairs always had two piles of clothes, one waiting to be washed, and one waiting to be put away. We were not educated; I was the only one of my five brothers and sisters that graduated from high school. We were not Protestant; we were Jewish, a minority in the predominantly Catholic towns and cities in the Boston area.

Ruth and her mother knew I was Jewish. I made no secret of it and it made no difference to either of them. The fraternity I joined was Jewish because, at that time, Jews weren't accepted into Christian fraternities. I could easily admit to being Jewish despite the fact that, in Boston, when I said that I was Jewish, I was treated by my classmates as if I had an incurable affliction.

Although I answered any questions that Ruth asked about my family, I was not very forthcoming. I was extremely reluctant to discuss my background and childhood with her or with anyone else. The truth was that I was embarrassed about my upbringing because I believed that everyone else in the world, except me, had normal families. I had no idea what normal was, but I was acutely aware that my family did not act the way other families did.

Now that I was in school and no longer living with my family, I wanted to desperately fit into Ruth's world. I was honestly afraid that Ruth would reject me if she ever learned about my upbringing. I was so concerned about my own family that it didn't dawn on me, until years later, that Ruth's family was almost as dysfunctional as mine.

I was just as curious about her as she was about me, but I was careful not to ask her questions that I wouldn't want to answer if she asked the same question of me. I relied on statements from her and her parents. They were both glad to talk about their daughter and, as a result, I learned more about Ruth than she learned about me.

In a way, it was funny. We both wanted to know about the other's upbringing but we each wanted to hide our own. Ruth was persistent in her questioning and she wanted a lot of details. I was more patient, just slowly gathering information and piecing the facts together. Neither of us was candid or open with the other. We both had family secrets that we were unwilling to reveal. Neither of us lied, but both of us avoided fully answering the questions.

After we broke up, I realized that not being open and honest with Ruth had guaranteed that our relationship would fail. My unwillingness to talk about myself was a mistake that I would live to regret.

It was only after we got back together again that we discovered that we had both been evasive about the details of our family life. We had hidden from each other and that meant that we had hidden from ourselves.

*** 

Ruth Ormondroyd was born in Wilkinsburg, Pennsylvania on February 11, 1929. When she was six years old, her father accepted a teaching position in the Engineering School at the University of Michigan and the family moved to Ann Arbor. The house Professor Ormondroyd bought on Copley Road was the only home Ruth knew in Ann Arbor. The family consisted of Ruth, her mother, father, and older brother, Edward. Edward was on the West Coast during the time that Ruth and I were going together so he and I did not meet until after Ruth and I got married in 1993.

Ruth and I were walking across campus about a week after we met when she said, "Jay, I want you to come over my house next Sunday afternoon and eat dinner with us. My mother and father would like to meet you."

I asked, "They won't mind me staying for dinner?"

"No, not at all. For the last few days I've been telling them all about you and they're interested in meeting you."

"If you've told them the truth, I'm done for. But, yes, I will be glad to come over next Sunday."

As I walked over to Ruth's house that Sunday I was nervous. It took less than five minutes to walk from the fraternity house, but that was long enough for me to envision my making a fool of myself in front of Ruth's parents.

Her mother and father were sitting in the living room when Ruth met me at the door and escorted me into the house. It was a large room, about thirty feet long, and her mother was at one end of the room and her father was at the other. Her mother, Mrs. O, as she insisted I call her, sat in an upholstered chair away from the walls. She stood to shake my hand when we were introduced. Mrs. O wasn't quite as tall as Ruth. She had short, blond hair, and her skin was tanned and a little leathery, the result of the constant sunbathing she enjoyed. She had large, square shoulders, an ample bosom, a heavy build, and she carried herself regally. Physically, she was a very imposing woman. I could easily picture her as a Valkyrie, wearing a helmet with a horn on either side, carrying a spear in one hand, and a shield in the other.

There was a table on the right hand side of her chair holding her books, her crossword puzzles, her drink, usually a gin and tonic, cigarettes, and an ashtray. She read avidly and could carry on informative conversations on many topics. She had a floor lamp over her right shoulder, and there was a huge Zenith console radio against the nearby wall. The radio had just been converted to receive the newly licensed FM radio stations, and she generally had classical music playing. Armed with her reading, her puzzles, her drink, her music, and her cigarettes, Mrs. O was totally self sufficient in the front of the room.

Professor O sat in the back of the room. His chair, a large wooden chair with an upholstered seat, a cushioned back and wooden arm rests, was located in one of the corners. He also stood to shake my hand. Professor O didn't make the same commanding physical appearance as his wife. He was thin and angular and he slouched as he stood. Until you noticed his eyes, always bright from the intellect behind them, his hawk nose was his most salient feature. Judging by appearances, it looked as though Mrs. O was the dominant character. However, looks can be deceiving. In his chosen field of work, mechanical vibrations, he was one of the most respected men in the world. Both the business community and his academic colleagues were constantly seeking out Professor O as a consultant. A brilliant mathematician, he became Chairman of the Engineering Mechanics Department with a Bachelor of Science degree as his only formal education.

To his right was a long table that covered most of the back wall; he kept an ashtray on the table's edge, next to his chair. Piled high on the table and also piled around his chair, were stacks of technical books, magazines, and treatises. With a floor lamp over his right shoulder, a drink near his right hand, and a cigar that he was always smoking, Professor O was totally self sufficient in the back of the room.

After a few visits, I came to realize that these were really their battle stations.

It was a pleasant visit. The four of us were on our best behavior and the afternoon and evening went quickly. As I was leaving, Mrs. O invited me to come back whenever I had free time.

After seeing them together a few times, it became obvious that Mrs. O and the Professor didn't get along. In their own stubborn, individual ways they fought like cats and dogs. They never raised their voices, as that would be impolite, but the cold contempt they felt for each other permeated their lives like the smell of cooking at a barbecue. Mrs. O had an active, agile mind and she possessed a very sharp tongue. She didn't suffer fools gladly, and she never made any attempt to hide her disdain of any one or anything she did not like. She would sit at her battle station, fortified with a drink, and fire salvo upon salvo of verbal abuse towards her husband.

In many ways, he was the typical absentminded professor. He wasn't handy around the house when it came to fixing or repairing anything. He would forget errands he had promised to run, and he was constantly misplacing either his glasses or his pen. He enjoyed bird watching and every weekend he would get up at the crack of dawn and go with his colleagues to various bird sanctuaries.

At home, Professor O was the target of almost all of Mrs. O tirades. He would sit at his battle station, shielded by his books, fortified with his drink, wreathed in a screen of cigar smoke that he knew she detested, and just attempt to weather the barrage.

Until Ruth and I broke up, I was in their home constantly and I ate with the family fairly often. Usually I would eat dinner with them on either Friday or Saturday night. Upon occasion, or for special events like a birthday, her mother or father would invite us to accompany them to their favorite restaurant, the Town Club. It was a private restaurant and open only to its paid members and their guests. Because it was private, the Town Club could serve liquor in its dining room. All the other restaurants in Ann Arbor were open to the public and only sold beer and wine. It was because of the liquor that the Town Club was the favorite restaurant of both of Ruth's parents. At least Mrs. O and Professor O could occasionally agree on small matters.

Once, at the Town Club, Ruth and I were the targets of Mrs. O's wrath. We were holding hands under the table and, when Mrs. O happened to notice, her temper flared. A very loud and unpleasant lecture on decorum and public manners followed. And while she may have been correct, her caustic speech for such a minor breech made the rest of the meal miserable for all of us. Professor O did not say a word, but he drank even more than usual that evening and I felt like joining him.

Wherever we ate, either at home or in a

restaurant, the atmosphere, at best, was stiff and cold or, at worst, frigid and nasty. Once in a while, when there was no sniping, the conversations were animated and interesting. Sometimes there was a foreboding quietness around the table, but the majority of the time, Mrs. O was angry about something. Her petty, childish behavior would have been comical except that it stifled any feelings of pleasure or joy for Ruth and me.

She would use Ruth to express her displeasure with her husband. "Ruth, please ask your father to pass the salt." Or, "Ruth, please ask your father to serve me a second helping of vegetables."

Professor O wouldn't respond to his wife, he would also use Ruth as a sounding board. In the past, when he had tried talking directly to his wife, he had been snubbed or berated. To avoid both, and to annoy his wife, he would hand Ruth the salt and pleasantly ask, "Ruthie, find out if your mother wants the pepper too?" Or, "Ruthie, find out if it's the peas or the beans that your mother wants?"

If Ruth had not asked me to always accept the invitations, I would have turned down some of them. I wasn't comfortable in that corrosive family atmosphere and I knew that Ruth was miserable. We never discussed it but I knew that the strained relationship between her father and her mother bothered her.

However, there was one family ritual that she and I both enjoyed thoroughly. I called it, "Professor O's benediction". At the end of most meals, especially when he had been drinking heavily, Professor O would say, "I ate too much, I drank too much. OY OY OY GEVALT. OY OY OY GEVALT. OY OY OY GEVALT." Mrs. O would swear at him for being such a damn fool and he would sit, puffing on his cigar, with an angelic smile on his face. Sometimes, when the spirit moved him after his wife's reaction, he would throw in an additional, "OY OY OY GEVALT."

When her parents were not together, they could each be friendly and inter esting. However, their years of marriage had tarnished any love, hope, or respect that they had originally brought to their union. They were just not suited to each other and neither would adjust. According to Ruth, all she could remember were the battles that went on between them, especially the caustic remarks of her mother.

Her parents had extremely different backgrounds. Her mother came from a very wealthy and socially prominent Philadelphia family; her father was the only child of poor English immigrants. But more important than their backgrounds was the fact that no compromise and no quarter had ever been given between the two of them. When they were together, in public or in private, Mrs. O was always on the offense and Professor O was always on the defense. They were a miserable, unhappy couple and that unhappiness radiated from them like heat from a wood stove.

After I saw how hardhearted and mean they were towards one another, I began to wonder about their private behavior towards Ruth. She didn't say much about her parents, giving me the same kind of answers that I gave her, although she did say that her childhood and her younger years hadn't been happy.

When Ruth and I were together with only one of her parents, I paid close attention to their conversations. I wanted to know how each parent treated her.

It was obvious that Ruth and her mother weren't close. Mrs. O was imperious and cold, never spontaneously hugging or kissing Ruth or even patting her on the shoulder. Mrs. O acted more like a queen, haughtily ordering a subject to do her bidding, than a mother talking with her daughter. Several times, I heard her tell Ruth that, when Ruth was born, she had wanted a boy. I couldn't blame Ruth for not wanting to talk about her mother.

Ruth and her father had a better relationship. They not only had a filial bond, but they had also banded together to weather Mrs. O's autocracy. Ruth was tolerant of, and amused by, her father. Their discussions were relaxed and their personal feelings were obvious. Yet, I got the impression that Ruth was unhappy with him because he had never interceded to defend her against her mother.

One Sunday, as Ruth and I were sitting together on the side porch of their house, I asked, "Ruth, will you give me a picture of yourself?"

"I will if you will give me one of you."

"That's easy enough to do," I replied.

Ruth went into the house, ruffling my hair as she passed me. She was gone for a few minutes and then came back and, without saying a word, handed me two photographs. One was her high school graduation picture. The other was a slightly out of focus picture of a young girl who was very plump. I could not identify the little girl, so I asked, "Who is this?"

"That's me when I was twelve years old. I haven't shown that picture to anyone before. I was very fat and I was miserable. I felt like I was out of step with the world and some of my classmates made fun of me. Finally, one of the doctors at University Hospital figured out that I didn't have a dietary problem, I had a medical problem. As soon as they started a different treatment, the weight began to come off. I never forgot what it was like to be ridiculed." Then she smiled. "Which picture would you like?"

"Oh," I said, "I'll be glad to take the graduation picture. I think that the newer model is an improvement over the older one."

Why Mrs. O took a liking to me was a total mystery. It may have been that I was different than the other men Ruth had dated and I amused her, or it may have been that my upbringing was foreign to her and I interested her, or it may just have been that she was genuinely fond of me. Whatever the reasons, she spent hours asking questions about my background and just talking with me.

Ruth occasionally got annoyed with me for spending so much time with her mother and she let me know about it. I grew to like Mrs. O. She could be nasty and domineering but she also had a quick wit and a marvelous sense of humor. I had never met anyone like her before and I found her fascinating. She amazed me more than she scared me. We got along well and that surprised Ruth.

She told me that her mother had always been condescending and not pleasant to her other boy friends. I could easily believe that. For the most part, Mrs. O treated me much better than she treated her own daughter. I never understood why.

***

My recollections of my own childhood are not sequential and straightforward. They are jumbled, skewed, and fragmented as if I was either trying to forget, or didn't want to remember, the details. Children need to have constant assurance that their world is level while they are growing. Without that assurance, they think that they are falling downhill. My world never felt level.

My full name is Jay Erwin Carp and I was born December 24, 1927. The doctor did not record my name until a few days after my birth and he got it wrong. My birth certificate has my name, incorrectly, as Joseph Erwin Carp. As a result, all of my legal documents and later, all my government clearances, list me as Joseph Erwin Carp, Also Known As (AKA), Jay Erwin Carp. To be dogged my entire adult life with an AKA because of a clerical mistake at birth is silly and I railed against it for long time until I realized that there was nothing I could do about it.

I was the middle child of five siblings. First came my older brother, Sheldon, who was called Buddy, and an older sister, Marcia. After me, there was my younger sister, Edna May, and my younger brother, Dickie.

My mother's parents came from Germany and settled in upstate New York. My birth certificate lists my mother's name as Annette Blumfield, and her birthplace as Pine Plains, New York. My father's death certificate has her name spelled as Annette Bloomfeld. My family seems to have problems with official documents. My mother had a sister who lived in the Boston area for a while when I was growing up. Her sister, along with her children, moved to Florida, I think, and I do not know what happened to them. I vaguely remember seeing my mother's father once when I was about four years old. He came to our house when we lived in Roxbury and slept in my room for a few nights. I don't remember ever hearing his first name and I have not seen or heard from my cousins since I was a youngster. That is all that I can recall about my mother's relatives.

On the other hand, we always lived near my father's parents, and I remember more details about them. My father's parents emigrated from Lithuania and settled in Boston. Their names were Ida and William and they both spoke heavily accented English. My grandmother's house was always clean, and the kitchen was the center of all family activity. Whenever we came to visit her, she would always pile food on the table for us. She would be upset and think we were getting sick if we didn't eat everything that she stacked on the table.

I don't think that she and my mother ever became particularly close, but she was always kind and loving towards us. I remember my grandfather as a quiet gentle person. Every fall, he would make small kegs of sour green tomatoes and half-sour pickles. I can still picture him shaking the spices and pickling ingredients off them as they came out of the brine; I liked their smell and their sour pungent taste. To this day I enjoy eating half-sour pickles and sour green tomatoes. It is odd how some memories become engraved in the minds of children.

Once, when I was in the fourth or fifth grade, I asked my grandmother about our family name. Some of my classmates had begun calling me Jay Crap, and I was convinced that my last name was the ugliest name in the world. She told me that she hadn't known my grandfather in Lithuania but she did know his family and that their name had always been Carp. I still believe it is an ugly name, but I have had so many arguments and fist fights because of it that, now, I wouldn't think of changing it.

My father, Benjamin, was born in this country along with his brother and two sisters.

He told me that he had wanted to go to medical school but, at the outbreak of World War I, he went into the navy. Upon being discharged, all of his plans changed after he met my mother who was working as a bookkeeper in my grandfather's firm. When they decided to get married he abandoned the idea of becoming a doctor and, instead, went into his father's wholesale fruit and produce business. Eventually, he left my grandfather's firm and went into business for himself.

From the time I was born, my father owned his own fruit and vegetable business. He always worked hard and a sixty or seventy-hour workweek wasn't uncommon for him. He was a good fruit and vegetable buyer but a terrible judge of personal character. He trusted everyone and, because of that, he lost all of his savings at least twice.

The first time, his partner embezzled a large sum of money from the business and then disappeared. The second time, he became a partner in a newly opened business that rebuilt automobile armatures and generators. The partner defrauded him and they had to close the business and dissolve the partnership. Within six months after the company folded, as World War II approached, his ex-partner got a government defense contract and reopened the business under his own name, leaving my father out in the cold.

Rather than declare bankruptcy, a disgrace in those days, my father worked tirelessly for years to pay off all of his debts. I didn't understand the importance of his honoring those debts until years later, and, when I did, I realized that my father was an extremely honorable man. I am proud of him not only for doing what he did, but also because he taught me that my word has to be my bond.

I must have been about eight or nine years old when my father joined the Masons. I had the impression that this was his escape from the crushing burden of running a business, working long hours, and paying back his debts. Whatever the reasons, he enjoyed belonging and he became both a Thirty-second Degree Mason and a Shriner.

My older brother, Buddy, also became a Mason and that pleased my father. I think my father was disappointed that I never followed their lead but, by disposition and experience, I'm somewhat of a loner. My fraternity was the only group that I voluntarily joined and even there I often felt out of place.

My childhood memories of my father are as thin and as transparent as a pane of glass. We five children seemed to grow up with only the one parent, my mother, ever being present. I remember my father as a quiet, harried man who avoided confrontations. He was either working, sleeping, or going to Masonic meetings.

I don't remember ever going anywhere alone with my father. I am sure we must have done things as a family because I recall seeing a photograph that was taken at Nantasket Beach, of my mother, my father, and all of my brothers and sisters, in bathing suits. Every year my grandparents rented a summer cottage in Nantasket, an ocean town south of Boston. My parents rented a flat for the summer, two years in a row in Revere, an ocean town north of Boston. Those summers stand out in my memories because the beach in Revere was made up of sea stones while the beach at Nantasket was sandy.

The price that we paid as a family, because my father was always working, was huge. Although we were a family by birth, we did not have a family circle. My brothers and sisters and I had to fight our own individual battles as best we could. We children each grew our separate ways, like weeds in an unkempt garden. There was no family unit to help keep us together.

My memories of my mother are much more concrete than my memories of my father. My mother was a pretty woman who had to bear the burden of raising the five of us. With my father being home so little, he was rarely involved with either our upbringing or our discipline. My mother made all the day to day decisions and she made them with love, not with logic. Over the years the stress must have taken its toll because she did not have the strength of character to rein in five children by herself. We grew up with as little supervision as any children were ever lucky enough to have.

There were mother and son memories that I can recall. I remember her taking me to see the Boston Braves play baseball and I am almost sure that Babe Ruth was in the lineup. I remember her driving us out to Norumbega Park, in Newton, to go on the rides. We would also visit a monument to Leif Eriksson that was along the Charles River in Norumbega Park. She would occasionally take us to a restaurant in Boston's Chinatown when she had some extra money.

However, my mother had a problem that had a lasting effect on all of our lives. She had a weakness for playing beano, which is what bingo was called in Boston. In retrospect, I believe that she must have been addicted to gambling. That is the only explanation that can describe her actions.

The three youngest siblings, myself included, would be left in our car for hours while my mother sat inside the hall, hunched over her beano cards. She was oblivious to her children and the rest of the world. In the summer we melted, and in the winter we froze. When she won we feasted, when she lost we fasted. Win or lose, on the way home we were always admonished not to tell our father where we had been. I couldn't understand why we were being left in a car for so long and why we shouldn't talk about it. I was always careful never to mention anything about my mother playing beano to my friends. I guess I wanted to avoid even more ridicule.

The results of her addiction rang through my childhood. I am sure that my father gave her a household allowance but nothing in our house ever ran on an even keel. Several times, our electricity, gas, and telephone services would be shut off until back payments could be made. Sometimes, our milk and newspaper deliveries would also be interrupted. I don't think that the water was ever shut off but it may have been.

Many times, our meals were adequate but sparse, consisting of bread, butter, fruits and vegetables. My father would occasionally ask, why aren't we eating any meat or fish and my mother would say, this type of diet is supposed to be healthier, or, the meat and fish didn't look fresh today. That would satisfy my father and the discussion would end. I never found out if he did not know, or if he just did not want to know, what was happening.

Compounding my feelings that my family had secrets that were shameful, was the fact that my family moved frequently while I was growing up. By the time I got to high school, there had been at least seven moves and there may have been more. All of our moves were within the Metropolitan Boston area, and sometimes, as in Brookline and Malden, we moved within the same cities. Because we changed houses so often, and had our utilities occasionally shut off, and from the look of the insides of our houses, I assumed we were poor. I had no measuring stick to know this, but I saw the more orderly households of my friends and, when I asked, they told me that they didn't move as often as I did. I didn't like the frequent moving because I was never able to keep friendships for very long.

From the time of my early youth until I left home to go into the army, the experiences and memories I had made me believe that my upbringing was entirely different than my peers. When I was small, almost all of my clothing consisted of hand me downs from Buddy. In a large family that is expected and I never gave it any thought, especially since all of my classmates were also wearing their older brother's clothes.

But, when I was older, sometime just before junior high school, I was much bigger than

Buddy was and my hand me downs began to come from my father's closet. The pants were too short in the legs and too big in the waist and everyone in school noticed the difference. They made fun of the way my pants fit and that really bothered me.

After I became aware of girls I got even more self-conscious. I wanted clothes of my own, so I once asked my mother for a new coat. She told me that she would buy me a winter coat, and she came home from Filene's Basement one day with one that fit me nicely. I was happy because it was attractive and warm and, with my brand new coat, my classmates would stop whispering to each other about my hand me downs.

I don't know what changed her plans. Perhaps she found that she needed the money to prevent a utility from being shut off. At any rate, before I even had a chance to wear it to school, she returned my coat and got her money back. She apologized to me, gave me an old coat that my father had worn, and told me that next spring she would get me a much better one. I was miserable.

The first party I ever attended was when I was in the sixth or seventh grade. Some of the girls in the class had organized into a group that they called the Crystal Club. They had invited several boys in their class, including me, over to a chaperoned party at one of their homes. These were all girls from well to do Jewish families and I felt that, for this party, I wanted something more than my usual hand me downs. My mother promised I would have a new outfit in time to go the party, but I never got the new clothes. She took me to a local shoe store and bought me a pair of cheap shoes that weren't my size. They hurt my feet and I thought that the oxblood color called attention to my big feet. Just before I left the house to walk over to the party, she pressed my only pair of pants. She told me that I looked handsome and sent me on my way. I knew that I wasn't handsome and I was troubled about what the girls would whisper about me. I felt completely out of place and, because I didn't know how, I declined all offers to dance. I was never more uncomfortable at a party than I was that evening.

Shortly after that, we moved again. My father had rented the end house in a row of three story townhouses. There were eight or ten of these houses and the neighbors could each sit on their own front steps and talk to the other neighbors without raising their voices.

After we moved in, I developed a crush on a girl who lived three doors away. I don't remember her name and I don't even remember what she looked like except that I thought she was pretty. I do remember that I liked seeing her and talking to her and that I wondered what her breasts looked like.

We lived there for only a short time when our mattresses became infested with bed bugs and they were constantly biting us. None of the neighbors had bedbugs, but we certainly did. They must have been in the mattresses when we moved because our mattresses were crawling with them.

To remedy the problem, every Saturday morning we would bring our mattresses into the third floor front bedroom, light some Paris Green candles, and then shut the bedroom door so that the fumes would fill the room. The Paris Green candles burned with a heavy, thick, sulfuric smoke that was supposed to kill the bed bugs. However, since we had to fumigate every Saturday, we obviously never got all of them. By late Saturday afternoon the candles would have burnt out and it would be time to put the mattresses back on our beds. Buddy would open the bedroom door, and, holding his breath, dash over to the two windows, open them, and dash back out of the bedroom. He would then slam the door shut. The dark, gray smoke would pour out of the front windows. After most of the smoke and the choking smell abated, all of the other windows and doors on the third floor would be opened to ventilate the entire floor. I don't remember how many months we did this, but it became a regular part of our weekend routine. Of course, we did not mention it to anyone because none of the family wanted the neighbors to find out about our shameful secret.

One day, I was sitting on the front steps eating a brownie that my mother had just baked, when the girl I had a crush on came over and sat down beside me. I offered her a piece of my brownie and she took it and started to bite into it. Suddenly, she turned, looked directly at me, and asked, "Jay, why does your house catch on fire every Saturday afternoon at four o'clock?"

I was absolutely mortified. No single question has ever shamed me as much as that one did. For years, the embarrassment of that moment has haunted me. Ruth was the first person I ever wanted to tell about my weekly fire, and, when I finally told her the story, I felt better. Now, I can not only laugh at that incident, I can even wonder what happened to the girl who asked me that question.

My self-doubts, my family's life style, and my inability to be comfortable around girls were not my only problems, nor even my major problem. At every school I attended, and there had been many schools because we moved so often, I had been the target of religious prejudice. I would do my best to avoid, or ignore, any confrontation but there were always a few boys who would taunt me. The more rabid of my tormenters would bump against me or try to push me down. Maybe it was because of my size, or my name, or maybe it was due to my hand me down haberdashery, but, whatever the reason, I was always taunted for being Jewish. For a long time I could not understand why I was being singled out for such derision. Although my grandparents were Jewish, my parents didn't celebrate any religious observances other than high holidays. Except for Yom Kippur and Rosh Hashana I was almost totally unscathed by formal religion until the time of my Bar Mitzvah. After that, when my father began to spend so much time at work, all religious observances disappeared.

As a child, I was told by my parents, with love, that I was Jewish, now, as a youth, I was being told by my peers, with hate, that I was Jewish. It made no sense to me that people who did not know me could dislike me.

When I told my father about what was happening to me in school, he told me that non-violence was the best way to defend myself. He said that there always were a few ignorant people who blamed everyone else for their own problems. He believed that a soft answer would usually turn anger away, and he advised me to ignore them and go about my business. And I, wanting to be a good son did exactly as he told me.

But I did have my doubts that his advice was doing me any good. By avoiding any confrontation and not defending myself I seemed to invite even more ridicule and abuse. The bigotry and the prejudice that I was subjected to left scars. I could not understand why I was ridiculed and why anyone would want to make me feel ashamed of my parents, my relatives, and myself. I had done nothing to them. I tried to be friendly and I was rebuffed; I tried to be aloof and I became the butt of venom and ridicule. I couldn't figure out how I was supposed to act and I really just wanted to be left alone.

I finally learned how to react, much to my delight, one day in junior high school. Just before the start of gym class, one of the biggest boys in the class started picking on me. He began by calling me names and swearing at me. When I paid no attention to him, he began to push me around. In response, I turned and walked away from him. But, the more I tried to avoid him, the angrier he got and the harder he would push. Even then, I still tried to walk away. He finally got so mad that he waved his finger in my face and said, "You Jews are the people who killed Jesus Christ. You bastards deserve to be punished." He pulled back his fist and punched me in the jaw. The blow threw my head back and cut the inside of my lip. I could taste my own blood. I had never been struck before and I was stunned for a second.

Then, I went absolutely berserk and, for the first time in my life, I fought back. I don't remember anything else about the fight until the gym teacher got between us and told me to stop before I killed him.

A tidal wave of elation engulfed me. I had thrown off my passive attitude and I had been the giver instead of the receiver and, despite what my father said, it was one hell of a good feeling. Although I had disobeyed my father I was not at all dismayed. Standing up to this bully made me feel like a man and, much to my surprise, I discovered that I enjoyed fighting.

From that day forward, I was not only left alone I was even grudgingly accepted by some of my former tormenters. I had learned a valuable lesson. The more you let someone bully you the more you will be bullied.

As I grew to physical maturity, I kept my thoughts and my feelings to myself. My social experiences had been painful and my problems, either imaginary or real, made me unsure of myself. I became wary. In an attempt to forestall anyone I had doubts about, I tried to discourage casual conversations. When I felt uncomfortable, in a deep voice, I would grunt, "Family motto. Big like bull, dumb like ox." Even though that discouraged most attempts at communicating, it also kept me penned inside my own corral.

After I entered high school, I began working almost full time in my father's store. Except during football season, when I played football, I would work every weekday after school and every weekend. World War II was being fought and there was a manpower shortage. I worked long and I worked hard and I did whatever I was asked to do. At that time of my life, I never questioned anything.

As soon as I graduated high school, I was drafted. It was 1945, and the Allies were beginning to win the war. During basic training I decided to go to paratrooper school and make a career jumping out of airplanes. Sometimes I pictured myself parachuting into Europe to fight the Germans and sometimes I pictured myself parachuting into the Pacific theatre to fight the Japanese. Where I landed wasn't as important to me as stopping the evil that was facing our country. I really believed that jumping out of airplanes would have been fun. Other than being a paratrooper for the rest of my life, I had no plans.

But none of that ever happened because I got rheumatic fever right after basic training and was confined to bed rest, in an army hospital, for six months. Because I was absolutely restricted to bed, I spent almost all my time reading.

I read everything in the hospital library and started to go through the books in the base library. It finally began to dawn on me that, because I was not going to stay in the army, I would need some kind of an education. The fact that the government would pay for it convinced me that I should go to school. Until that time, I'd never thought about going to college. Truthfully, I had never really thought about much of anything.

I was the only member of our family to graduate from high school and, after I was discharged from the army, my father was surprised that I didn't want to stay with him in the fruit and vegetable business. He would say to me, "You send a horse's ass to college and all you get back is a horse's ass covered with a sheepskin." I was not sure whether or not he was referring to me, but I did know that, even if I couldn't explain it to him, I wanted something other than the fruit and vegetable business.

I enrolled at the University of Michigan using the GI Bill to pay for my schooling. I tried out for football and played on the freshman team as a defensive lineman. I had hoped to earn a varsity letter and that being a member of the "M" Club would help me land a job. While I was on the freshman team, Phi Sigma Delta rushed me, thinking that having an athlete in their fraternity would be a feather in their cap. Even though I had been a loner most of my life, I joined because I was homesick, I was by myself, and I wanted friends.

Everything went awry towards the end of my freshman season. We had practiced for weeks as a team and we were finally scheduled to scrimmage against the varsity. I hurt my ankle during the scrimmage and I went to have the trainer look at it. He was busy with the varsity, so he glanced at it quickly, told me that it was a slight sprain, and recommended that I stay out of practice and walk on it for a day or two. Even though the pain was excruciating, I did what I was told, and when I returned, they discovered not only a broken ankle, but also that the walking had strained the ligaments. I was in a cast for months and my ankle was never strong enough to play football again. I would never have become an All-American, and maybe not even a starting lineman, but I probably would have earned a varsity letter by my senior year. Not to have done so was a disappointment for me.

Once I was in the fraternity, I was surprised by the affluence of all the other members. Most of them had large allowances and they spent money without giving it any thought. It was as much a reflex for them to buy whatever they wanted as it was for me to breathe. It was a lifestyle that I had never seen before and I was uncomfortable with it. I liked a lot of my brothers and I was close to a few of them, but I thought that the majority of them placed too high a value on material goods. I couldn't keep up with them financially, nor did I try. There was a difference between their attitude and mine and I got the feeling that most of them were snobs. Inside myfraternity house, I felt as out of place as an Eskimo in Africa. If my fraternity brothers were velvet, than I was burlap.

By the time I met Ruth, I was paying formy room and board by washing pots and pans in the fraternity kitchen. My pocket money came from the GI bill, from selling my blood at both the U of M and St. Joseph hospitals, and from the few dollars my family could occasionally send me.

\*\*\*

As our junior year ended, I was unsure of what I was going to do during the summer. Ruth was planning to work in the Admissions Office of the University full time until the fall semester. She had worked there the previous summer and they were glad to have her back. I had no spcific prospects, and I did not want to leave Ruth. On the other hand I felt an obligation to go home to see my parents and work in my father's store. By this time all of my brothers and sisters had gone from the house, so my mother and father were alone. I wanted the opportunity to tell them about Ruth.

Although Ruth was hoping I would stay with her in Ann Arbor, she didn't try to influence my decision. After wavering back and forth, I finally decided that I should return to Boston. I did want to help my parents as much as I could and I did want to see them. They were sending me what they could afford and I was glad to get the money. It was a difficult decision, but I would be returning in a few months and Ruth and I would be together for our senior year. Reluctantly, we said our goodbyes. We promised not to date anyone else, and to be faithful until we were together again in the fall.

It turned out to be a terrible summer for me. When I got home, I found that my mother and father had moved, once again, and were living in the Back Bay area of Boston. My father and a new partner had opened a fancy fruit and vegetable store on Massachusetts Avenue, near

Boylston Street. They combined their two names and called the store, "Malben's." The store specialized in quality produce, imported cheeses, and fruit baskets.

My parents lived in an apartment house that was less than two hundred yards from the store. The apartment was on the third floor and it was hot, dirty, and cramped. It had no air conditioning, no view, no light, and, I thought, no hope. I slept on a mattress on the floor in a cramped bedroom and ate my meals, usually by myself, by opening the refrigerator door and grabbing.

My daily routine began the moment I got there. I worked long hours at the store, six days a week. I would drive a truck into the wholesale market before dawn, load it with fresh fruit and vegetables, and return to the store. Once the truck was unloaded, I would work until the store closed at 8:00PM. Most of my Sundays were spent sleeping. It wasn't the hard work that bothered me particularly as I was used to the long hours. It was the heat that I disliked. It was an exceptionally hot summer and the apartment was stifling. The bathroom was small and grungy and my showers didn't seem to wash any of the dirt off me. I felt hot, sweaty, and filthy all summer long.

Worse than the discomfort was the fact

that my parents and I never talked about anything important. I searched for a chance to sit down and tell them about Ruth and my studies but we all seemed unavailable. My mother had a part time job and, when she wasn't working, she was out playing beano. That apartment was so cheerless that I didn't blame her for staying away. My father's schedule was like mine, so he was either working or sleeping. He had aged considerably since the last time I had seen him and he was physically exhausted. He seemed to shy away from any personal discussions and he was no longer even interested in attending Masonic meetings. If I hadn't overheard him telling his customers that I was the son that was going to the University of Michigan, I would not have known that he was even aware that I was going to school. It was a classic case of a son who didn't know how to talk and a father who didn't know how to listen. We all lost out that summer.

My nights were what I dreaded the most. Almost every evening, after I fell asleep, I had a nightmare that left me shaking and frightened. I would dream that Ruth had talked her mother and father into driving her to Boston to surprise me with a visit. They found the apartment and knocked on the door. Wearing only my underpants, and not expecting to see them, I would get out of bed and open the door. The three of them would take one look at me, one look into the apartment, and then they would turn around and, without saying a word, they would walk away. My dream always ended at that point and I would wake up, soaked in sweat.

I missed Ruth and I wrote and called her frequently, but my conversations were short and my letters were skinny. I told her I loved her and missed her and that I was anxious to get back to Ann Arbor. I tried to avoid mentioning anything about my family because I did not want her to find out about my living conditions.

On the other hand, Ruth was as cheerful and talkative as usual. She told me that she loved and missed me and she could hardly wait for me to return to Ann Arbor. She knew that I wasn't upbeat and kept asking me if everything was all right. I assured her that nothing was wrong; it was just that I was tired from my long hours of work and that I missed her. Those, by themselves, were absolutely true statements. However, since I did not want to tell her anything else, I ended up by telling her nothing.

My summer of horror lurched along and, finally, it petered out. I said goodbye to my mother and father with mixed emotions. I would miss them, but not the conditions under which they lived. I left without ever discussing their future plans or my future plans, or even telling them about Ruth. I should have tried harder to talk with them, but at the time, I did not know how to open up and express my feelings.

When I got back to Ann Arbor, I dropped my belongings off at the fraternity, freshened up, and ran over to Ruth's house. The front door was open and I knocked hard on the screen door. In a few seconds she appeared at the door in a green smock; her face was moist with sweat. I was stunned anew by her beauty. The summer sourness that had pickled my thoughts for all those weeks began to evaporate the minute I saw at her. All I could do was stare at her and say, "Hello, sweet Ruth."

She immediately started fussing with her hair. The humidity had tangled it and made it curly. "Damn you Jay Carp, why didn't you call me before you came? I have been ironing and I am a sweaty mess. Come here, I've missed you."

I opened the screen door and entered the house. We embraced in the vestibule and were kissing each other deeply when I heard a distinct, "Ahem." We jumped apart and I turned around to see her mother glaring at us.

Mrs. O said, "I see that you're back from Boston, Jay."

"Yes, and hello Mrs. O", was all I could lamely say.

Much to my surprise, she offered her cheek for me to kiss She said, "Well, plan on staying for lunch." Then she went into the living room leaving Ruth and me alone to talk to each other. Luckily for me, we were so busy talking about our feelings for each other that Ruth never pressed me for any details on my family.

If my miserable summer had taught me anything it was that I desperately loved Ruth. The only joy I had had all summer was when I thought of her and the things that we had done together. Now that I was again beside her, my only goal was to make her happy. We were both in love and committed to each other.

A week after I returned from Boston, just before our senior year was to begin, I decided to ask Ruth to wear my fraternity pin. It never occurred to me that Ruth wouldn't accept it. I was sure that she felt the same way about me as I did about her.

When we first met, she had told me that she had been pinned twice before but that she had broken off both relationships. She hadn't gone into any detail. Later on, after we became serious about each other, Ruth told me what had happened.

The first time was when she was a senior in high school and her boyfriend was a sophomore at Michigan. She was flustered when he asked her to take his pin and she didn't know how to say no. She took it and, after less than a week, she gave it back and told him that she was sorry, but that she just wanted to date. Their relationship cooled and ended shortly after that.

The second time was more complicated. Just after her she enrolled at the University, she started dating a senior in medical school. They had fun together, and enjoyed their dates, and, after a few months, he asked her to take his pin. She accepted the pin without thinking of all of the consequences. After she started wearing it, her boyfriend became very possessive. If he found her talking with another man, he became angry. Worse for her, was that he started to make sexual demands. When he tried to feel her up, she slapped him and returned the pin. For weeks he called, apologizing and saying that he was sorry, and that he would never do it again. It took Ruth a long time to get him to stop calling, and an even longer time for her to get over the bad feelings and memories of that episode. When she told me those stories, Ruth said that she was never going to accept a fraternity pin, or an engagement ring, unless she was in love.

We were sitting on the porch watching the fireflies sending their messages to each other in Morse code. Ruth was smoking a cigarette and we were both drinking from open bottles of beer.

In the darkness I leaned over and put my Phi Sigma Delta fraternity pin in her hand.

She asked, "What is this?"

"My fraternity pin."

"Jay, you know how I feel about accepting a pin, don't you?"

"Yes, Ruth, I know. This is my commitment, I love you."

"And I love you Joseph Erwin Carp. I am happy to wear your fraternity pin."

We kissed and held hands for a few minutes. Ruth took another swig of beer and then asked, "Why did it take you so long to offer me your pin?"

I laughed and asked her, "Now that you have it, how soon will it be before you give it back to me?"

"Never," she replied, and thumbed her nose at me.

Our senior year was even more idyllic than our junior year had been. We were as inseparable as cream in coffee. On class days, we would meet at the bus stop, go to campus, and spend the entire day together. On the days we had no classes, I would be at her house, talking with her mother and father, until she and I left and went somewhere. When we needed it, Ruth would borrow her mother's car and drive us to wherever we had to go.

## The Gift of Ruth

That time was a happy, carefree, innocent time for us. We were young, in love, enchanted with life, and completely oblivious to the possibility of problems. Neither of us had worries or thoughts of what our future might hold. We lived for the happiness that each day brought us and assumed that we were living in an open-ended cornucopia of joy.

It was only after we graduated that we began to lose each other.

\*\*\*

From the time that Ruth and I had first met, until we both received our degrees in 1950, we had lived in a college environment. We were isolated from the stresses of normal everyday living with all of its money problems and hard decisions. In a sense our love, which was as rich and sweet as maple syrup, existed in a vacuum, free from all turmoil.

I didn't realize that the feelings that flowed so freely between us needed infinite protection. But love will evaporate and disappear when it is neglected or taken for granted. I was too young to know how to take care of our precious commitment. Ruth and I always talked only about the present; we never discussed our future. The result was that we watched our love bubble, then fizzle, and eventually vanish, like an Alka Seltzer in water. I had no idea how to stop the process.

The changes in our lives, after we graduated, had immediate effects upon us. The first change was that Ruth, upon getting her degree, started working full time in the Admissions Office. Her summer work had impressed the Dean of Admissions, and he wanted her to join his staff.

I was another matter entirely. When I entered Michigan, I had no idea of what I wanted to study or what I wanted to do for a living. I enrolled in the Liberal Arts School and got a degree in English. I had never given any thought about what I was going to do after I graduated. The result was that I had a degree, a lot of knowledge, some intelligence, and no idea of how to earn a living. Along with my personal doubts was the fact that I was totally unprepared to enter into the commercial world.

Secretly, I had thought that I wanted to be a playwright. Outwardly, I said I wanted to go into advertising. Realistically, I knew absolutely nothing about either. I compounded my problems by never discussing my goals or plans with anyone because I was afraid of ridicule. So, I hid my ideas from everyone, my advisors, my fraternity brothers, and even from Ruth. My capabilities never caught up to my ambitions. It was too late for me before I learned that if a person lacks the courage to state his goals, he also lacks the strength to meet his goals. When I graduated, I really wasn't smart enough to find my way out of a glass telephone booth.

Four or five of my fraternity brothers offered me jobs in their family businesses. I looked into one or two of these opportunities but their family attitudes convinced me that the offers were more of a charitable deed than a commercial need. I bristled at working for anyone under those conditions, so I did not pursue their job offers very hard.

After I got my degree I should have gone into Detroit to find a job, but I could not bear the thought of leaving Ruth. Instead, after a few part time jobs, I ended up in a downtown Ann Arbor stockbroker's office working as a clerk for minimum wage with the possibility of being trained as a stockbroker.

My new expenses left me with almost no spending money. Ruth volunteered to share the costs of our dates and that made me feel like a beggar in Baghdad. Ruth was happy with her job prospects. I felt trapped.

Another change was that we were no longer living near each other. I had moved out of the fraternity house into a rented room downtown and we did not see each other nearly as much as we had when we were going to school. We needed to make arrangements just to meet, and, with both of us working and without a car, getting together wasn't easy.

But the biggest hurdle weren't the changes themselves, it was that I did not know how to handle the changes. I was a boy in a man's frame. I didn't know what to do with our problems, so I paid no attention to them, hoping that they would go away. I think that, to some degree, Ruth did the same thing. This was where the crack in our relationship first appeared.

When we first met, we had each talked endlessly. Our days weren't long enough for us to express our thoughts and opinions. While we were together our experiences were common and we shared them joyfully. Now, we each spent our days apart from each other. New concerns, and the changes we were seeing in each other, seemed to dry up our spontaneous conversations. We were no longer effervescent.

Neither of us understood what was happening. We were not happy but we both shied away from discussing the changes. I was hesitant because I didn't know what to do and Ruth was waiting for me to take the lead. It was a sure formula for failure.

To complicate matters even further, sex began to become an issue. Up until that point, our kissing had been more friendly than deep. Ruth did not tell me, and I would never have asked, but I was sure that she was a virgin. She was reserved and, although she liked jokes about sex, she would sometimes ask me to explain them to her when we were alone. I was so intoxicated with her that I didn't try to get intimate. Often, and innocently, we held hands, embraced, and kissed. While our relationship was built on closeness, camaraderie, and courtship, sex never was an issue. I suppose that we thought we would explore it after we were married.

As our relationship began to change, we slipped into different patterns without even realizing it. With less in common, and less to talk about, we began to snuggle more often. Being young and healthy we soon started French kissing along with fumbling, fondling, and petting. I started to like it very much and looked forward to it; Ruth started to like it very much and that concerned her. Neither of us said a word about what we felt and our heat actually began to widen our rift.

Our relationship faltered and failed slowly from the time we graduated in June until early the following summer. It was then that Ruth told me of her plans to take a two-week vacation on Cape Cod with a girl friend of hers from the Admissions Office. The minute she told me of her plans, I knew that when she returned we would break up. The months of worry about us, about money, and about what I should do, convinced me that we were through.

The two weeks she was gone were absolute hell for me. I could not sleep, I could not eat, and all I could do was berate myself.

Ruth returned to Ann Arbor on a Sunday afternoon, and when I called to speak to her, she told me she was very tired and that she was going right to bed. She avoided all contact with me the next week, but she did invite me over her house the following Saturday morning. When I arrived, she was sitting on the front steps waiting for me. I sat down beside her and she told me that she knew this last year hadn't been good for either of us, and she felt we should break up. She said it was the hardest decision that she had ever made, but she thought it was for the best.

I sat there in sorrow and in silence. I couldn't disagree. We were spinning away from one another. I couldn't offer any solution so I had to accept her judgement. We sat there, holding hands with tears in our eyes. We would be silent and then we would talk for a while. Ruth wanted to give me back my fraternity pin, but I refused to take it. It meant nothing to me any more; it was a trinket for which I had absolutely no use. What had been between us would never be duplicated, so I did not want it.

Ruth asked me what I was going to do and I told her that, outside of moving to Detroit and getting a different job, I really didn't know. I stood up and we said goodbye.

Our beautiful interlude was finished. The lights were turned down, the music was silenced, and we each traveled our separate paths.

For many years after that, I kept thinking of the words of John Dryden;

*"None but the brave deserves the fair."*

## SUMMER

After driving almost twelve hours, I arrived at my motel in Ypsilanti around four o'clock in the afternoon. When I got through the Windsor Tunnel, heading into Detroit from Canada, I got lost and I drove around a city that seemed war torn and violated. Entire city blocks were burnt, as if they had been fire bombed. Rubble and charred lumber sat piled up on empty lots, mute testimony to the hopelessness and indifference that was gripping the city. Houses were boarded up, abandoned, and left with no protection against dope peddlers, drunks or vandals.

Detroit held little resemblance to the lively place where I had worked so many years ago. This was my first trip back into downtown Detroit since leaving the area as a young man and the blight depressed me. When I finally found the freeway to get to Ypsilanti I was tired from driving, and uneasy by what I had just seen. There was a long distance left to travel and, this first leg of the trip between Westboro, Massachusetts, and Santa Maria, California, had not begun pleasantly.

Finding the motel where Ruth had made

reservations for me was no problem as her instructions were easy to follow. However, nothing in the Ann Arbor/Ypsilanti section around the motel looked even vaguely familiar. If it were not for my memories, I would have sworn that I had never been in this area before. I registered at the desk and made sure that the reservation that Ruth had made for me was for Friday night, Saturday night, and Sunday night. Then I went to my room, unpacked, and rinsed my face. After that, I called Ruth at her place of work.

"Huron Valley Consultation Center," is the way she answered the phone.

"Hi, Ruth. This is Jay. I just arrived at the motel a few minutes ago."

"You're a little late aren't you?" she asked. "I was beginning to get concerned."

"To tell the truth, Ruth, I was beginning to get a little concerned myself. I made a wrong turn out of the Windsor Tunnel and I found myself taking a tour of downtown Detroit."

She chuckled. "I'll bet that shocked you. Listen, I'm a little busy right now, I have got to go. Your motel is almost directly across the street from my office. I'll come over right after I finish work, sometime after six o'clock. Will that be OK?"

"Sure, Ruth, that'll be fine, I'll be here. I am in room 127. Looking forward to seeing you." With that I hung up the phone. Because I wanted something to do, I showered, changed into fresh clothes, walked around the lobby, came back to my room, and, finally, sat in a chair. What was running through my mind was that, after forty years, I was going to see Ruth again. It was something that I hadn't imagined happening and I had no idea what to expect. After everything that had taken place in my life during the past year, I was trying to neither look ahead nor look behind. All I wanted was just to cope with the present.

\*\*\*

We had been living in Westboro when Virginia, my wife of thirty-seven years, died suddenly, and unexpectedly, at our daughter's apartment in Raleigh, North Carolina. Virginia had arrived in Raleigh on a Saturday afternoon, and passed away in her sleep on Sunday morning. I was totally unprepared. I put my wife on a plane at 4:00PM one day, and, at 6:00AM the next morning, I got a phone call from our daughter saying that she was dead.

After bringing her body back to Massachusetts, none of my three daughters could attend the burial service I held for Virginia, so I planned a memorial service at a later date, when all my daughters could attend. That service was held six months later. After the burial, I went to my boss at General Telephone and Electronics (GTE), where I had worked for thirty years, and I asked to be laid off. I didn't want to work any more because I felt that there was nothing left to work for. After a few months, GTE complied with my request, and I was put on layoff status.

My last field assignment had been as GTE Field Manager at our office at Vandenberg Air Force Base. While Virginia and I were in California, we bought a house in Santa Maria, a town just outside of the air base. When we returned to Massachusetts, we rented an apartment in Westboro, planning on returning and living in Santa Maria after my retirement in a few years. When I stopped in the Ann Arbor area, to see Ruth and her mother, I was on my way to the house in California.

Over the years, Mrs. O and I had kept up an infrequent correspondence. I never knew why she wrote, and I never thought much about it. I would get an occasional letter from her and I would try to answer her within a few weeks. Months would then go by, I never kept track of the time, and then another of her letters would show up. She would ask my opinions about political matters, politicians, or events that interested her. Her letters only concerned her affairs, she had not written about Professor O until his death and there was never any mention of Ruth.

As a matter of fact, I didn't have any idea that Ruth was in the Ann Arbor area until I got a letter from her, saying that her mother had just been put in a nursing home. Her mother had asked Ruth to write me and inform me of her change of address.

Ruth wrote that her mother's eyesight was failing and Mrs. O wanted all her mail sent to Ruth who would then read it to her. Ruth's letter to me had been sent to the house in Santa Maria about a year and a half after I had moved back to Massachusetts. That I actually got it was unusual as the post office forwards mail only for a year after an address change.

I showed Virginia the letter and then answered it. Mrs. O had met Virginia after she and I had gotten married. After Virginia died, I wrote Mrs. O a letter about her death. On my way to Santa Maria, I planned to stop off in Michigan to see Mrs. O. She was in her eighties, in poor health, and wouldn't be around much longer.

What I was anticipating was a calm weekend visit with an old friend and an old flame and then continuing on my way to California. Is it a blessing or is it a curse that humans can't predict the future?

Feeling a little restless, I went to the mirror to look at myself. The reflection showed a big man, sixty four years old, scarred by time, overweight by about twenty-five pounds, and with a full head of hair that was rapidly turning gray. I muttered to myself, "I sure as hell look my age."

Just then, there was a gentle knocking on the door. I walked over and opened it and saw a tall woman with short, gray, blond hair. She stood there staring at me as much as I was staring at her. Was this Ruth? The years had taken their toll but they had not taken her beauty. Oddly enough, her right hand was raised and closed as if she were ready to knock again.

We looked at each other as if we were trying to bridge the years since the last time we had met. Unconsciously, we extended our arms and were holding each other's hands.

"Hello, Ruth," I said.

"Hello, Jay. Is your room okay?"

"The room is fine, Ruth, but the motel doesn't have a restaurant or a bar. So come on in. We have to decide what to do this evening, and where to eat."

Ruth entered, put her purse on the edge of the bed, sat down in one of the stuffed chairs, and said, "I have no idea what your plans are for the weekend, but the best time to visit my mother is right now. Parking at the nursing home can be a problem on the weekends. And as far as eating goes, there are plenty of good restaurants in this area, depending on how much you want to spend."

I agreed that we should visit her mother first. I had not specified anything in particular for this weekend. Being in Massachusetts, I had no idea what would be going on in Michigan. I had asked Ruth to make herself available and find out what was happening in Detroit and Ann Arbor. I figured that, after I arrived, we could decide together what to do. We talked briefly about a few restaurants and I asked her about a couple of names that I had seen in the yellow pages.

"Well, let's go see your mother first, and we can pick a restaurant later. Why don't we leave your car here and we can go in mine, there's no reason to take both cars is there?"

So we started over to her mother's nursing home in my automobile. As we exited the parking lot, Ruth told me to turn right on Carpenter Road. I did and when we very close to the intersection of Carpenter and Washtenaw, Ruth said, "Jay, you can either get in the left lane and turn left, or stay in the right lane and go straight. Either way will take us to her nursing home."

This caught me off guard as I was almost through the intersection when she gave me those options. I had no idea how to get to the nursing home and I was depending on her for directions. I quickly looked out of my mirrors and made a sharp left turn. Immediately, I heard the squealing of tires and a horn blaring.

Ruth then said, "You really should get into the right lane because we have to get onto 23 going north." I cut into the right lane immediately, and two more drivers honked their horns because I came close to sideswiping them. We had no more close calls on the way, but I was annoyed about the way Ruth was giving me directions.

As we drove on route 23, the traffic thinned and Ruth and I had a chance to talk. She said, "Jay, I don't understand why you and my mother have been writing to each other all of these years. How did that ever get started? I asked her about that when she wanted me to write and tell you she was in the nursing home. She never really gave me an answer. Can you?"

I thought for a while and I could see Ruth watching me as I searched my memory. Finally, I replied, "I'm not sure I really know, and it may be a long winded answer. A few years after you and I broke up, I returned to Ann Arbor to go to engineering school. I met Virginia, we married here, and my first two daughters were born here. We were not in close contact, but your mother did see Virginia and my daughters occasionally.

"My guess is that when Virginia and I left this area, we initially kept in touch with your mother during the Christmas season. Virginia was a great one for sending Christmas cards. The more I think about it the more I would be willing to bet that that is how our correspondence started. Our letters were always sporadic; your mother would write and I would answer. Then time would pass, I would get another letter, and I would answer. And so it went for years and years."

Ruth asked softly, "Did she ever mention me in her letters?"

I looked at Ruth quickly, chuckled, and replied, "That is a question that I can answer without any hesitation. She never mentioned you, or your brother, and she only mentioned your father when he died. Outside of the changes of address on the envelopes, she never mentioned moving. She stuck strictly to her own health and general comments about what was going on in the world. Now that I think of it, that is a little strange.

"I had not heard of you, or about you, since you married and left Ann Arbor. Until I got your letter, telling me your mother was in the nursing home, I did not even know that you were living in Ypsilanti. How long have you been living here?"

"I have lived in the house I am in for almost thirty five years. We bought it when Mike first got out of the Navy and went to dental school," she replied. By this time, after more directions on roads without much traffic, we had arrived at the nursing home.

Before we went in, I said to Ruth, "Did you know that I visited your mother on my way through Ann Arbor about eight or nine years ago?"

"Really? No I did not know that. What was the occasion?" Ruth asked.

"We were driving from Massachusetts to California. There was myself, Virginia, my daughter Julie, who was divorced, an Old English Sheep dog, and a cat. We were all on our way to my new job at Vandenberg Air Force Base. Virginia had wanted to make it to Chicago to see her best friend but we had only gotten as far as Ann Arbor. We came over to the Glacier Hills apartments and visited with your mother late in the afternoon.

"In a way, it was a funny kind of visit. We had the cat and dog in the car because we did not want to leave them behind at the motel. So, while we were in your mother's apartment, Julie kept checking on them through the window and even though we were six floors above the parking lot, Julie kept talking to them through the window. That annoyed your mother. We only stayed about an hour before your mother started to get tired and cranky so we said goodbye and the next morning we left for Chicago. Your mother never told you?"

Ruth replied, "No, but that is not unusual. Until my mother broke her hip and had to leave her apartment for the nursing home, I saw her as little as possible. She and I never got along. She did not like me and I hated her when I grew older. I perform all the duties required of a respectful daughter but I can't get over her treatment of me when I was a child."

That was a total surprise to me. I had not guessed the depth of her animosity towards her mother. I immediately wondered about her use of the word hate. She didn't like her mother and she may even have really hated her, but, as I subsequently saw, she did take care of her as well as any loving daughter would.

My visit with Mrs. O was disturbing. The last time I had seen her she was frail and old but she had been in complete control of all her faculties and she had been ambulatory. Now, she was in a semi-private room in a nursing home and, like all rooms in all nursing homes, it was too small, too cluttered and it had too much furniture. On her bedside stand, which had been pushed to the foot of her bed, were discarded wrappers, paper cups, and a food tray left at supper but not yet taken back to the kitchen. The air in her room smelled stale from old food, old body odors, and old people.

Mrs. O was lying on her back under a sheet with her eyes closed and her arms folded on her chest over the sheet. She looked nothing like the woman I remembered from her apartment. She was a wrinkled skeleton with wild, uncombed hair. Her muscles had atrophied and she could no longer take care of herself. Her mind wandered and returned only to wander again. It was hard to tell when she was lucid and when she was inside of herself, divorced from the rest of the world.

"Mother, Jay is here to see you," Ruth said loudly. She had to speak in a near yell because her mother was hard of hearing. She repeated herself three more times before her mother gave any indication that she had heard Ruth.

Mrs. O finally opened her eyes. She raised her right arm slowly, motioned with her right hand, and let her arm fall back to the bed. "Hello," she croaked.

"Hello, Mrs. O," I said as I leaned over and gave her a kiss on the cheek. "How are you feeling?"

"Oh, not very well," she murmured in a tiny voice. "I can't see very well and I don't hear very well. So I just lie here and wait."

"Mother, would you like a gin and tonic?" Ruth asked her.

Mrs. O replied, "Oh, that would be nice."

Ruth beckoned at me with her head and we left the room and went to the nurse's station. She asked the duty nurse to unlock a cabinet that contained Mrs. O's gin, tonic water, and a plastic bottle of lime juice. Ruth fixed her a drink in a plastic glass and returned the makings back to the cabinet.

Ruth held the drink while her mother-sucked noisily on a straw. We made as much small talk as we could with Mrs. O while she drank her gin and tonic, but Mrs. O didn't do much talking. I am not sure she heard us. When she finished her drink, we told her that we would be back to see her on Sunday, before I left town. I couldn't tell if that statement had registered with her or not. We left the room and as soon as we got out of the front door I took several deep breaths of fresh air. I could clear the smell from my lungs but I could not clear the thoughts from my head.

"My God, Ruth," I said. "That is awful. How long has she been like this?"

"My mother fell and broke her pelvis just over two years ago. She absolutely refused to try any rehabilitation, so she became bedridden. Since then, she has slowly cycled downward and ended up in this nursing home over a year ago. I visit her twice a week and I try to get my daughters to visit her when they can; but it is really difficult to get them to come over here and see her. It is depressing to visit her. As you saw, it is hard to carry on a conversation."

"I can't blame your daughters, it is pretty grim in there." I replied.

Before I started the car we continued our discussion about restaurants. I asked her about one called "Robbie's at The Ice House". The name caught my eye when I was browsing the yellow pages before Ruth arrived.

"That is a very expensive restaurant, Jay," Ruth said. "There are plenty of other places that won't cost nearly as much."

"But is it any good, Ruth?" I asked.

"Oh yes, it is very good but their prices are very high. There are less expensive restaurants available," she replied.

I decided that we would eat there. "It sounds like a good place to eat. The name interests me, the cost doesn't. It is a good thing that we are not going Dutch Treat, isn't it?"

Ruth laughed. It was the light laughter of

a young girl not the throaty chuckle of a matron and it totally surprised me. For the first time, Ruth smiled as she said, "Well, I am glad that I am not paying. I do thank you, but I want you to know that there are cheaper restaurants where we could go."

She continued to look at me with a pleasant expression on her face. This was the first softening of our mutual wariness. "Perish the thought," I told her. "If we are not satisfied, we will go to McDonald's later and get a real meal. In the meantime, point me at this joint."

I drove into downtown Ann Arbor following Ruth's directions. The only problem we had was when she did not give me enough notice to change from the left lane to the right lane to make a turn. I came close to hitting another car and I was blocked off from getting into the correct lane. We had to continue for another two blocks before I could circle around and come back. By this time, I was irritated that I had come close to having another accident because of her directions.

"Robbie's at The Ice House" was not busy, which was a good thing for us because we took hours to talk, only occasionally eating and drinking. We started with before-dinner drinks and then continued with appetizers, entrees, desserts and coffee. Everything we ordered was excellent and as expensive as Ruth had predicted. She grumbled about the prices a little, but she had to admit that it was a nice restaurant.

We were busy talking and trying to catch up on the intervening years since we had parted. Ruth seemed less reluctant to talk about herself-than I was, so she began first to tell me about her past. She talked rapidly, using short sentences.

She had married a little over two years after we broke up. Neither her father nor her mother thought much of her husband. She said it was the first time they had been agreed on anything important in years. Her husband, Mike, was in the Navy when they married, and he was trans-ferred to San Diego after the wedding. When they returned to this area, they bought a house in Ypsilanti, with a down payment she borrowed from her parents. Her husband enrolled in den-tal school and, when he graduated, he opened a practice in Ypsilanti.

It was during his last year in dental school that their problems, simmering since the start of their marriage, really boiled over.

Ruth quickly found out, while they were in San Diego, that Mike not only drank to excess, he was a womanizer. His drinking and womanizing went out of control while he was going to den-tal school. Mike purposely went out of his way to have an affair with one of her best friends in their neighborhood. When Ruth found out, she was furious and deeply hurt. It marked the end of their husband and wife relationship. After he opened his dental practice, Mike began to come and go as he pleased and within a few years their marriage was a wreck. Ruth kicked him out of the house, finally got a divorce, and became a single mother with three young girls. Mike paid neither alimony nor child support, and he had even tried to mortgage her house, without her permission, after she got it as part of the settlement. Eventually, due to malpractice, Michigan barred him from practicing dentistry.

When Ruth finished her narrative, she looked at me and said, "When I was young, I knew so much, and now, years later, I know so little. Have I become smarter or dumber? I do not know. Either way, I am anxious to hear about you and your life."

The beginning was easy enough to outline for Ruth. After she and I broke up, I went into Detroit and worked for almost three years. While I was working in Detroit, I became interested in engineering and I returned to Ann Arbor and enrolled in engineering school. While I was going to school, I met Virginia and we got married. Two of my three daughters were born at the U of M Women's Hospital.

I worked for General Telephone and Electronics for over thirty years in military electronics, mostly on the Intercontinental Continental Ballistic Missiles, Minuteman, Peacekeeper, MX, and Rail Garrison. I did a lot of traveling to the missile sites. Sometimes my job was exciting, sometimes it was demanding, sometimes it was frustrating, but it hardly ever was boring and I thoroughly enjoyed my work.

When I said that, Ruth looked at me in surprise. She said, "Jay, I just can't picture you in that kind of work."

"Ruth, don't shoot the messenger," I laughed. "Personally, I never believed in the 'Nuke them all' philosophy. But, don't forget that your father, who was a very peace loving man, worked for Admiral Rickover, and, although he hated Rickover, he did like the work he was doing on nuclear submarines." She thought that over for a while and agreed with me.

We chatted for a few more minutes and, finally, Ruth said, "You know, you have not said a word about either your marriage or the death of Virginia. Are the memories of her passing still painful for you?"

I sat there quietly for a while, as I really did not want to talk about my marriage. Finally, I said, "Virginia's death was so sudden and so unexpected, that it didn't make any sense to me. I still don't understand what happened.

"Virginia and I had been married for thirty seven years when our middle daughter, Julie, was confined to bed for the last trimester of her pregnancy. She lived in Raleigh, North Carolina. When Virginia found out that Julie was going to be bed ridden, she wanted to fly down and take care of her. Virginia had been a registered nurse. I had no problem with her being gone that long and we both agreed that a mother really should be with her daughter at a critical time like that.

"But I did have concerns about Virginia's health and her general well being. Years before she had had cancer and, after that, she had suffered a heart attack. Virginia was a fretful woman who constantly said she was tired. She was always worried about the future and, for some odd reason, she had a terrible fear of ending her life as a bag lady.

"However, her routine examination at the Lahey Clinic, which she had less than two weeks before she went to North Carolina, found her physically in good shape. There was no medical reason she should not go.

"So, I made reservations for her to fly from Boston to Raleigh on a Saturday. Immediately after the arrangements were made her mood changed. Virginia seemed happy that she was going to be with Julie when her new grandchild was born. She didn't say anything about being tired and she began to give me lists of things to do, and instructions to follow, while she was gone. I took the week before she left as a vacation week and we spent the time going on day trips to New Hampshire and Maine. To reassure her about our future, I showed her what I expected our income to be after I retired. We spent a quiet, pleasant week together. She seemed free of her normal worries and anxieties.

"She was quiet while we drove to Logan airport early Saturday afternoon. Just before she boarded the plane, she turned and came back to where I was standing and looked at me. She gave me a quick peck on the cheek and said, 'Jay, thank you for letting me help Julie. I love you.' Then she got on the plane.

"I don't know why, but I keep remembering her thanking me for letting her go. Virginia didn't have to thank me, Julie needed her help and Virginia had worked as a delivery room nurse for years.

"I called her that evening, sometime after supper. She told me that she was a little tired and that she was going to go to bed early. She said that she would call me tomorrow and that I was not to worry, Julie and she were both fine.

"At that time, Julie's husband, Michael, was working the midnight shift, and when he came home he would sleep on a sofa so as not to disturb Julie. So, Virginia and Julie went to bed together. About six o'clock Sunday morning, the phone rang, and when I answered it Julie shouted, 'Dad, Mama is lying in bed with me and I think she is dead. What am I going to do?'"

I stopped talking. Like all lengthy marriages ours had had good times, bad times, and ups and downs. Virginia and I had been through it all and our marriage had endured. But, during the last nine or ten years, our marriage had slipped from an equal partnership between husband and wife into a relationship in which I was more of a caretaker. It had become a marriage of rote, not a marriage of passion.

I didn't tell Ruth any of the details of my marriage until later. However, I was obsessed by my marriage. Since Virginia's death, I had been wrestling with my conscience and with the negative emotions of grief, rage, shame, and sorrow.

I had been punishing myself with recriminations for almost a year. I could have been and I should have been, a more caring and nicer person, and now it was too late. I sat there, staring at my plate.

Ruth sat quietly. After a while she leaned across the table and patted my arm. We both sat in silence. "Well, so much for our pasts," Ruth said in a low voice, "What are your plans for tomorrow?"

We talked about it, and decided to go to the Ann Arbor farmer's market in the morning and the Michigan State Fair, in Detroit, in the afternoon. That would pretty well fill up our entire day and since it was getting near midnight, we decided to leave and get some rest. When we started to drive back to the motel, Ruth again began giving me options as we got close to intersections. "You can continue straight, or you can get in the right lane," she said.

After I nearly got sideswiped again, I decided that I had to say something. I was more than a little annoyed. I didn't want to start an argument but I did want her to know that I wasn't happy with her directions. "Ruth, I don't know my way around, and I will rely on your judgement. It will be easier if you pick out the best way to go and just tell me how to get there. That way, we stand a better chance of getting where we want to go without having an accident."

She apologized, and I told her it was nothing major, and from then on, she gave me simple directions. We drove to her car, she got into it, and then I followed her to her house in Ypsilanti. By doing that, I would know how to get there in the morning. I joined her at the front door and Ruth invited me in, but I declined; I was honestly tired. I told her I would call in the morning. I opened the door, saw her in, and went back to my motel.

I lay in bed and I felt a little depressed. Seeing the condition of Mrs. O, talking about Virginia's death, and even thinking about the way Ruth gave directions, distressed me. Luckily, I fell asleep quickly and spent the night untroubled by dreams.

*** 

When I arrived at her house early Saturday morning, Ruth was sitting in a chair on her porch waiting for me. We ate a leisurely breakfast at a local restaurant and we lingered over coffee, talking seriously about nothing and enjoying ourselves. When we got to the farmer's market it was noisy, crowded, and fun. We walked along the stalls, asked the farmers about their produce, joined in on the constant group conversations that begin, pass information, and then dissolve as quickly as they start. We bought fresh fruits and vegetables and baked goods. On the way back to her house, while I drove, Ruth fed me pieces of the cookies we had purchased.

When we got inside her house I was totally taken aback. It was dark, shabby, cluttered, and threadbare. The green carpet was worn and had holes that Ruth had tried to hide by covering them with scatter rugs. All of the furniture had multiple cigarette burns both on the fabric and on the wood. There were stacks of newspapers, magazines, books, and clothes all around. When I saw the inside, I began to realize how hard it must have been for Ruth to be a single parent, make a living, and raise three daughters.

When we got to The State Fair, I paid our admission fee and then bought a lot of ride tickets because Ruth said she enjoyed the rides. We walked around looking at all the exhibits and we found ourselves in a large building that was filled with pens that held small male goats. I was totally amazed; I had never seen such small animals with such huge gonads.

I looked at Ruth, she looked at the rams, and then she looked at me. She smiled and then she giggled. "I am not a connoisseur," she said, "but those are really big balls."

I shrugged my shoulders and replied, "Beats me."

We both laughed, and walking arm in arm, we went through all the exhibits. Late in the afternoon, we stopped and had a beer. As we drank, I asked her, "Are you ready for the rides, or would you rather eat something first?"

"To tell you the truth, Jay, I am a little hungry," Ruth replied. "But will you be all right, eating first, and then going on the rides?"

I stupidly tried to be funny and bragged,

"Oh heavens yes, I will be fine, I am almost chemically inert."

We both had another beer. I had a large kielbasa and Ruth had a slice of pizza. I had a third beer. After we finished eating we went on the whip.

The ride had not even been spinning a minute before Ruth looked at me and asked in alarm, "Jay, are you all right?"

I wasn't. For the first time in my life, the ride was making me queasy. My stomach was flipping and I was not sure whether or not I would throw up. It was the longest five minutes I had ever spent, and through it all Ruth held my hand tightly and talked to me softly, telling me to keep my eyes closed and breath deeply.

When the ride finally stopped, she pulled the safety bar back, helped me out of the seat, and walked me to the nearest bench. I sat there dizzy, nauseous, and ashamed. Ruth disappeared, and shortly she came back with a can of Coke, and she told me to try to take little sips from the can. I did what she suggested and, in a few minutes, I began to feel a little better.

"Are you all right? Has this ever happened to you before?" Ruth wanted to know.

I replied, "No, this has never happened to me before and I feel goddamn stupid and goddamn embarrassed."

Ruth held my hand and looked me in the eyes. "Jay," she said, "Stop that. You do not have to apologize to me for not feeling well. It could have been a bad Polish sausage or it could have been anything. And it really doesn't make any difference what caused it." Then she smiled. "Or maybe you got sick because those rams had such big balls. In any case, let's just sit here until you feel better."

After about ten minutes my dizziness and nausea disappeared and I began to recover. Both of us thought it would be wise to call it a day and head back to Ann Arbor. As we walked to the entrance I tried to give away all the ride tickets that we had not used, about twenty dollars worth. I had a lot of trouble disposing of them. When a couple with young children came by, I would explain why I was not going to use the tickets, and I would ask them to take the tickets and use them free of charge. I guess the parents were frightened; no one would accept the tickets. Finally, a family, with two youngsters, reluctantly accepted them. On the drive home Ruth said that it was sad that people were so afraid of each other that they wouldn't even accept free ride tickets from strangers.

When we arrived back at Ruth's house she invited me in. The lamps she turned on had small wattage bulbs and they did not cast much light. I was sure that was part of her never-ending fight to cut costs. She asked me how I felt, and, when I assured her I was fine, she mixed us each a drink. She had a gin and tonic I had a bloody Mary. We talked continuously about our kids, our jobs, and ourselves; we were knitting together the frazzle of loose ends that the years had frayed.

"Jay," Ruth finally asked, "do you like California?"

"Oh yes. I love the sunshine. It invigorates me. The area I live in, Santa Maria, is about fifty miles north of Santa Barbara and the mornings generally start off cloudy or foggy. But by mid-morning the sky is clear and the sun shines the rest of the day. For me, the sun just seems to take the aches and pains out of life. You lived in California, what did you think of it?"

She said, "I enjoyed it but that was many years ago. Mike was in the navy and we were living in San Diego. My first daughter, Robin, was born in California. I went back to San Diego three years ago because my bowling team was in a tournament out there and I visited Coronado. I was so disappointed at the changes to that beautiful area that I cried. I guess you can't ever go back." She was quiet a moment and then she asked, "What are your plans when you get back to Santa Maria?"

"I have absolutely no plans," I replied. "My furniture is in transit from Massachusetts to California. The house is much too big for one person. Two of my daughters live in North Carolina and the other one lives in Texas. Eventually, I guess, I will sell the house, but I am not sure. I have no plans. What about you?"

She laughed as she answered, "That's easy. Things aren't nearly as tight for me as they once were, but my financial advisor says that if I want to travel when I retire I will have to work until I am at least seventy-two. So, barring my making a fortune by gambling, I will be working for another eight or nine more years. There are so many places that I want to see." She paused for a second and then said, "That's long range. Closer at hand, what do you have in mind for tomorrow?"

"Nothing really," I responded, "I would like to visit your mother and say goodbye; but I have nothing else in mind. Have you any suggestions?"

She hesitated a few seconds and then she asked, "Well, would you object to my introducing you to my daughters?"

I was a little puzzled by her question. "Ruth, why would I object?" I asked her. "I think that it would be nice to meet them. Though I am curious if you have told them anything about us."

"No, not really, hardly anything at all," Ruth answered, "But I had to say something to explain why I would be busy this entire weekend and probably wouldn't see them. I just said that I was seeing an old friend from college days and, when they found out it was a male friend, they got very interested."

"Well, I can't blame them for that. I am sure that we will be able to fit them into our busy schedule," was my response. I looked at my watch and was surprised to find that it was after one in the morning. I really didn't want to go but I figured I should. I finished off the last of my drink and stood up.

Ruth said, "I am enjoying myself, Jay, you don't have to go unless you want to."

"Ruth, I'm also having a good time. If you don't mind, I would like one more drink and then I really should be going."

We drank our drinks and began talking about the people we had known and the things that we had done so long ago. We were once again inhaling perfume inside the bubble of happiness. Time stood still and yet it went by so quickly.

Finally, I said "Ruth it is almost four in the morning. I think you should go to bed and I should go to bed." I still really did not want to go, but I figured I should offer.

Ruth walked me to the door and we stood facing each other. I was not sure whether to kiss her or not, when Ruth, in her own direct way, solved the problem. "Jay," she asked, "Don't I deserve a little sugar?"

I held out my arms and she came quickly into them and we kissed. Gently, at first, then deeply, and finally, passionately. We rocked back and forth. Ruth broke away, and breathing heavily, she said, "Old people are not supposed to act this way."

"Listen, Ruth," I said. "There is something I must tell you. I think—."

Then I paused. I waited for about ten seconds, and then continued. "Think? No, that's just plain bullshit. I do not think, I know. I love you."

Ruth blurted, "Jay, don't say that. We haven't seen each other in years. How do you know? How can you be so sure?"

I laughed. "I don't know how I know. How did I know the first time? I haven't the foggiest idea of how I know. What I do know is that I love you. I also know that I am not afraid to tell you. Don't you feel anything, anything at all?"

She nuzzled against me, and said, "Oh, Honey, of course I feel something. But I don't want to be disappointed again and I don't want to analyze it. I just want to enjoy it."

She came back into my arms and we embraced again. When we stopped to catch our breaths, she had a little smile on her face. She took a firm hold of my hand and said, "Let me show you the rest of the house." She led me into the bedroom.

***

Sunday didn't go as either of us had thought it would when we discussed it after we got home from the State Fair. When I woke up on Sunday morning, we were nestled together like two spoons. I had to go to the bathroom, and that presented a problem because her double bed was against one of the corners of her small bedroom and I was next to the wall. I was wondering about sliding down to the foot of the bed, slithering over the hope chest, and getting to the bathroom that way, when Ruth woke up. She turned around, looked at me, smiled, lifted her face to mine, and gave me a kiss.

"Good Morning, Lady Bug," I said, and then gave her a kiss in response.

"Good Morning, Honey," she replied as she lazily nestled back against me. "Lady Bug? Why did you call me that?"

"Absolutely no reason at all," I answered.

"I love you and that was the first thing that

came into my mind. You are a lady. If you don't like it, I won't call you Lady Bug again."

She lifted her face from my chest to look at me as she asked, "Oh no, Honey. I like it. Have you ever called anyone else Lady Bug?"

"Never, never, never, never. And I hardly ever use the word never," I replied.

"I like that," she said, "that's nice." She put her arm across my chest and rested her head on my shoulder. We lay there for a while, blissful, and, despite being unclothed, somewhat bashful.

Ruth said, after a while, "I am going to call 911. There is a naked man in my bed."

"Listen Ruth, if you will let me by you, I can use the bathroom and solve the naked man in your bed problem," I said.

"Such a gentleman, but what about me? Don't I get to use my own bathroom?" She put heavy emphasis on the "I" and the "my own."

"Go ahead, Ladybug. I will wait."

Ruth became very serious. "Honey, if you need to, you go ahead."

"Listen, if I wait for you and you wait for me we will both end up wetting the bed. For goodness sake go first. All I ask is that you hurry as fast as you can."

"OK, I am going, Jay. Please do not look," she said as she got out of the bed.

I did not understand her morning modesty after our midnight madness, but then I didn't have to. If she didn't want me to peek, I wouldn't peek. When she was through in the bathroom, I gathered up all of my clothes, went in, cleaned up, and dressed.

Ruth was standing by the dining room table waiting for me. On the table, cluttered with piles of books and newspapers, were two cups of coffee. She came into my arms and snuggled against me. "I am sorry, but it is instant coffee. That is all that I have. I can give you sugar and skim milk, if you take it, and I can make you some toast if you are hungry."

I hugged her and kissed her hair. "Ruth, Ruth, Ruth," I replied, "I take my coffee black, no sugar, and I am not the slightest bit interested in food." The tone of my voice, or the way I spoke must have caught her attention, because she pulled herself away and stared at me.

She asked me seriously, "You aren't sorry about last night are you?"

I thought about that for a second because I was not at all sure what she meant. I decided that whatever she meant didn't make any difference to me because there was absolutely nothing that I was sorry about. I laughed and said, "Ruth, I have found you again, I have found love again. I am not sorry about anything that happened last night. As a matter of fact, I was hoping to repeat last night's activities."

"Me too," she replied as she snuggled back against me. "But sit down and drink your coffee while it is still hot. We have to talk. You have got to tell me what your plans are."

I sat down and tasted the coffee; it was awful. I had made plans before I arrived, but now I needed to make new ones. Everything was up in the air, and in technicolor, like a fireworks display. I said, "Ruth, I was hoping that you would want to discuss your plans with me."

She looked at me and her lovely face was so somber I thought she might have been close to tears as she replied, "Honey, I am not trying to hide from you. I have exactly the same feelings you do. I just want to be careful, if I can. But I can't make my plans until you tell me what your plans are. After all, you are the one who owns a house in California and you are the one who is leaving tomorrow morning to drive to that house. So, you tell me what kind of plans I can make?"

And damned if I didn't have to agree with her. All of my arrangements had been made on the basis that, when I arrived in California, I would be single and without any attachments. I shook my head and smiled ruefully.

I said, "Ruth, you are absolutely correct.

The ball is in my court. But I had no idea what you would do to me when we met. At my age, I had not expected to fall in love again. And to fall in love with the same woman who was my first love is a miracle. I feel like I felt so many years ago, the very first day I ever saw you. Only this time I am not going to lose you."

I had to stop for a while because I was getting misty eyed. The combined memories of last night and forty years ago were catching up to me. We held hands for a while and then I continued, "My new plan is very simple. I will drive to California and be there to meet the furniture when it arrives. I will put the furniture in the house just as I had previously planned. Now though, instead of living in Santa Maria, I will put the house up for sale and come back and live happily ever after in Ypsilanti.

"And while I do these things, I will have to call my daughters and tell them of my change of plans. Will they ever be surprised."

Ruth's voice was loud as she said, "Jay, you can't do that."

"And just why can't I do that?" I asked.

Ruth quickly responded, "Because that's crazy, that's why."

"I have never claimed that I am not crazy. Right now, I am not only crazy I am also crazy about you. All that I want is to be with you, and

I can't focus on anything else. So, let's change the subject for a while.

"I would like to go back to my motel room to shave and get a change of clothes. Why don't you come with me and we can sit in their hot tub and talk more about this?"

Ruth thought this was a good idea, and we did get to the hot tub but it was not a direct route. When we got to my room, Ruth suggested that we clean up by taking a shower together. Showering with someone was something that I had never thought of, or done, before, but I catch on quickly and I agreed.

Ruth wouldn't get undressed until after I was in the shower. When she entered, we got wet, we kissed, we soaped each other, and we got horny. We had to rinse and dry ourselves so we could get into bed and have sex, an admission that our bodies were no longer as lithe and limber as they once were.

When we finally got to the hot tub, we were the only people in it. It felt good to sit in the hot water while it circulated around us. It certainly was relaxing; I almost fell asleep and my mind started to wander. All of a sudden I started to chuckle. Ruth, who had been sitting there with both her eyes shut, opened them, and asked, "What are you laughing about?"

"Ruth, you may not believe me, but I never

heard the thunder."

"Jay, what are you talking about?"

I replied, "What am I talking about? I am talking about you and me, me and you. Whoever said that lightning never strikes twice in the same place? I was struck twice and, both times, I never even heard the thunder. Either that or you are a witch feeding me secret potions. Ruth, I love you, I adore you. I want to marry you."

Ruth squeezed my hand and smiled, as she said, "Jay, will you please be sensible? I don't even know if I will ever see you again after this weekend is over. I thought that is what we came over here to discuss."

"First of all, Ladybug," I said, "I am being sensible, very sensible. I want to be with you. There is nothing more important for me than to be with you. And once I realized that, everything else falls into place. I will sell the house in California and we will live together here in Michigan. You and I have a lot of catching up to do."

She shook her head. She said, "We haven't even been together forty eight hours. How can you know what you feel? How can you be so sure?"

"I am not sure of anything except that I love you. It doesn't make sense but it doesn't have to make sense. Love is the fourth dimension. How do I know I love you? My eyes tell me, my heart tells me, my soul tells me, my gonads tell me. The only answer I can give you is that I want to be with you. Now you tell me what you want to do."

Ruth sighed. "I don't know, Jay, everything is happening so rapidly. I don't want you to go but I know that you have to. I want you to stay but I don't want to make a commitment. Everything happened so quickly, I just don't know. You're not disappointed with me are you?"

"No, Ladybug, I am not disappointed in the slightest. You are correct about this happening quickly. Trust me, though, I know that you love me. You just don't make decisions as quickly as I do. We will do just fine. Relax, and enjoy the ride. Our life together is going to be fun.

"What I am curious about though, is what do we say to your mother?"

Ruth splashed water on me and laughed. She looked at me and said, "Jay, I don't want to tell my mother right now. I don't want to tell anyone right now. I am not trying to hide anything. It's just that I have been alone for so long that I want to savor this moment in secret for just a little while. When you come back, we will tell everyone, but for the time being, let me enjoy my happiness quietly. Is that all right?"

Whatever Ruth wanted would be fine as

far as I was concerned. "Of course it is all right. All I wanted to know is what we were going to tell your mother. The simple answer to my question is that we will tell her nothing."

We lolled in the water for about an hour until a family of four came to use the hot tub. We returned to my room and showered together, without taking a sex break of any kind, got dressed, and visited Mrs. O. This time, Ruth's mother was almost entirely withdrawn inside herself, so there wasn't much conversation. We couldn't even get her interested in the pieces of cantaloupe that we brought her or in a gin and tonic. Considering what we were not going to tell her, it was probably just as well that she did not respond to us.

After our depressing visit, we went to eat at the Gandy Dancer, a restaurant housed in the old Ann Arbor train depot where I had arrived the first time I came to Ann Arbor. We ate leisurely. As we sat, full of food, full of ourselves, and full of each other, Ruth said, "Don't order any dessert."

I had not even gotten that far yet and I was too full to think about it.

"Why?" I asked.

She leaned towards me and whispered, "Because I am horny as hell and I want to go home."

"OK. But at least let me pay the bill first so that we can get out of here without being arrested."

Ruth replied, "Jay, nobody likes a wise ass."

When we returned to Ruth's house we went into the bedroom, got undressed, and went to bed. Unlike the other two times we started slowly. We lay there kissing, touching, and feeling each other softly. She told me what she liked and I told her what I liked. As we each got more excited, our movements got faster, we rubbed harder, and we got more vocal. We were feverish. We mated and writhed as one. We each chanted our own litany of ecstasy. Ruth moaned, over and over, "Oh Dear God, Oh Dear God, Oh Dear God." I grunted repeatedly, "Oh Jesus, Oh Jesus, Oh Jesus." We both climaxed and lay spent, panting, sweating and happily satiated.

After our breathing became normal, Ruth snuggled against me. I cocked my head so that I could see her face; I enjoyed just looking at her. She smiled at me and then frowned. She said, "Honey, this is crazy, this is absolutely insane. It is unseemly that a woman of my age suddenly gets horny all the time. For years, I have gone without sex and I have tried to put all thoughts of it out of my mind. Then you return, and now that is almost all I can think about. Am I turning into a nymphomaniac?"

At first I was going to reply, "I hope so." But as I watched Ruth, I could see that she was concerned, almost worried, over her display of physical passion. Now was not the time to try to be amusing, Ruth seemed so vulnerable.

After a while, I answered, "No, Ladybug, you are not a nymphomaniac. We are both just catching up. Even if you won't put it into words you really are telling me that you love me. What do you think?"

She must have been comforted by that thought because she snuggled a little harder against me. "Maybe you are right." She lay there for a while, and then continued, "I went to my bridal chamber a virgin. Mike always accused me of not being very good, or very interested in sex. He might have been correct but he was very abrupt and not very gentle. He said that it was my attitude that made him stray. As our marriage disintegrated we became more incompatible. He began to drink more heavily and screw every female he could, and I tried to stay away from him as much as I possibly could."

She raised up, kissed me on the lips and sighed, "And now I can't seem to get enough of you." Then she laughed and asked, "You are not slipping me drugs are you?"

She then became serious and said, "Honey,

I have to ask. Should I be concerned about getting AIDS?"

Well, I thought, That's an honest, straightforward question. She was so open and so candid that she deserved absolute honesty from me. I knew that it had not been easy for her to tell me about herself; I felt I owed her the truth. I looked directly at her. "Ruth, you do not have to worry about catching AIDS. I have not been sexually active for years. You stand a much better chance of getting pregnant than you do of catching AIDS.

"This is painful for me. I have never talked about Virginia and me before to anyone, but I guess we were as mismatched as Mike and you. Virginia and I had no premarital sex. After we were married I quickly found that her views on sex were entirely different than mine. Once, I told her that I wanted to eat her and she got furious. She told me 'Absolutely not. Only animals do that type of thing; good Christians do not do that'. I had never thought about it before, but it was hard for me to think of myself as an animal."

Ruth kissed my cheek. "Honey, I would like to try whatever you want to do. All I ask is that you be gentle with me." She thought for a while, and then asked, "Jay, were you ever unfaithful to Virginia?"

I waited so long to answer that Ruth asked, "Did you hear me?"

I sighed, and then answered, "Yes, I heard you, but the answer is difficult for me to tell you. I was unfaithful once. It occurred while I was living and working in Maryland while my family was still living in Massachusetts. GTE had laid me off in 1970 and that was a bad time to be out of work in New England. There were no jobs available in my field and, to make ends meet, I ended up with two full time jobs working 16 hours a day because I had to earn enough money to pay the bills. I worked in a factory in North Attleboro making dynamite cans on the midnight shift and then I drove a dump truck for the Foxboro Highway Department during the day. Virginia went back to nursing and she hated her job. I worked those two jobs for thirteen months. Finally, I got a job offer with a laboratory in Silver Spring, Maryland, to work on the Polaris ICBM carried on the Navy nuclear subs.

"Virginia and I discussed the job offer and we both agreed that I should take the job even if it meant splitting up our family for almost a year. This was at the time that Cynthia and Julie were both in high school and we didn't want to interrupt their education in the middle of the school year.

"I took the job and moved down to Maryland. For the first three months I drove the four hundred miles from Silver Spring to Foxboro every Friday, and then I drove back every Sunday.

"During this time, things were bad between Virginia and me. I sent every penny home that I could and, with her working as a registered nurse, there should have been enough money to cover our expenses, but she was always distressed. Every letter she sent was full of complaints about her job, unhappiness that the family was split, and worry about our bills. I understood her feelings but I was doing what we had agreed on. When I asked if she wanted to move down to Silver Spring sooner, she refused. Months of these letters along with the bad weekends that we had wore away at both of us.

"Virginia was miserable and there didn't seem to be anything that I could do to satisfy her. It wasn't until years later that I realized that the stress she was under began to change her. All I knew was that I used to look forward to receiving letters from home, but once they were delivered, I dreaded opening them.

"To answer your question, I met a very lovely divorced woman and I had an affair with her for about three months. I thought of getting a divorce, not so much to change partners, but to get out of the hell that I was going through. I thought about divorce very seriously but I just couldn't do it. When I told my lady friend that I was not going to get a divorce we both agreed to go our separate ways. Right after we stopped seeing each other GTE got in touch with me in Maryland, asked me to come back to work, and I returned to Foxboro."

Ruth asked me, "Jay, if you were both so miserable, why didn't you get divorced?"

"Because I couldn't walk away from the mess that I helped to create. First, I had to consider my three daughters. They were in their early teens and I didn't feel they should be punished for their parent's problems. Even a dysfunctional family is better than no family. I brought them into the world and I had responsibilities to raise them.

"And then there was Ginny. The strain of my layoff started her downhill mentally and she began to go to pieces. In her agitated state a divorce was the last thing in the world she would be able to cope with. I had taken a marriage vow the same as she had and I had a responsibility to keep my word. Whatever was wrong with our marriage couldn't have been all her fault. It wouldn't have been right for me to bail out and leave just because the marriage was not all that I wanted it to be.

"I am not proud of that time. I made errors and mistakes and I was not as patient with Ginny as I should have been. Yes, I had an affair. I never told Ginny, and that is all I want to say about it for a while."

We lay there, each of us thinking about what we had been through and wondering about what our lives might have been like if circumstances had been different. That type of thinking is a useless exercise because it never changes the past and it never points to the future. I gave it up, shook my head, and nuzzled Ruth.

"What?" she asked.

"Would you care to screw?"

She laughed, "Silver tongued devil, you should have been a lawyer. Honey, I am a little sore; my boobs are not used to so much attention. Would you be angry with me if I asked for a rain check?"

"No, I wouldn't be angry with you, Ruth. I'll give you as many rain checks as I can get printed. As a matter of fact I am not even sure whether I am bragging or not. My instrument is not used to any attention either, so I don't know whether I could get another erection. This golden age stuff is not all that it is advertised to be. I don't know about you, but I definitely have some physical limitations."

We giggled, then we snuggled and snoozed.

We were content. Just before dawn, I got up to return to my motel room to clean up and check out.

Ruth got up when I did and put the teakettle on the stove to boil some water. We were drinking instant coffee when Ruth casually asked me, "When does your furniture arrive in California?"

"I have been promised that it will be delivered a week from today," I replied.

"You said that you planned on driving five days; if your furniture is going to be there in seven days, you can stay in Ypsi for two more days. You can check out of the motel and move in here. That will be fun, won't it?" Ruth was grinning as she spoke.

"Ladybug, I can't stay. I am going to visit someone in Arizona."

Ruth stopped smiling. I could see the anger rising inside her. Her voice was not pleasant when she said, "You what?"

I repeated, "I am going to visit someone in Arizona."

"'Someone in Arizona,'" she mimicked. "When you say it that way it has to be a woman. You bastard. You dirty son of a bitch. You are going cross country with your thing going up and down like the needle on a sewing machine."

Ruth was furious and she was hurt. I am

sure that she felt that she had been betrayed.

I was totally stunned by Ruth's reaction. And she was completely wrong in what she was thinking. Then I felt badly. The last thing in the world I wanted to do was hurt Ruth. I had just found her again and I didn't even want to leave. But all of my travel plans, and the delivery of the furniture, had been made long before I left Massachusetts. If Ruth had not been wounded so deeply, what she was thinking would have been almost humorous.

She was out of line in believing that I was working my way across the continent pollinating all of the senior citizen rosebuds. I had never contemplated entering into a cross-country screwing contest. I knew she was misinterpreting my motives, but I also knew that her anguish was genuine.

"Listen to me, Ladybug, and listen to me well. You are wrong in what you are thinking. I made all my arrangements for this trip months ago. It never occurred to me that anything would happen between us. This woman that I am going to visit is almost a total stranger to me. She was a friend of Virginia's; they knew each other long before I married Ginny. Even before you came back into my life, I wasn't the slightest bit interested in her. She has been married and divorced at least three times. I would be wary of

114

someone like that and I have no intention of getting involved. I met her once, for a few hours, maybe thirty years ago. She and Virginia kept up a correspondence for years. All along I have thought of this simply as a courtesy call on behalf of Virginia.

"Ladybug, she means nothing. I will be back because I want to live the rest of my life with you. Don't make it any harder to leave you than it is now.

"Two things I can easily promise you; I will be good and I will be back."

Ruth didn't say a word she just sat there. I finished my coffee, stood up, and told her I would return after I loaded the car and settled the motel bill.

Then, I kissed her on the top of her head and walked out the door.

*** 

When I pulled the car into the driveway an hour later, Ruth was sitting on the front steps waiting for me. She walked over to the car and, when I got out, she put an arm on each of my shoulders and looked straight into my eyes.

She said, "Honey, I am sorry for being such a bitch and losing my temper. Words are hard for me to say sometimes. But I do truly love you

Jay, and, now that I have told you, I don't ever want to lose you. I've been worried about your trip and the possibility of your having an accident. I guess my concerns carried over when I heard about that woman in Arizona. I want you back with me."

She rested herself against me. After a moment, she kissed my cheek, smiled and added, "That is something that you never saw before, but I do have a temper. Is my tantrum about you driving off going to drive you away? Please come back to me."

Although I wasn't happy, I felt better about leaving. We were meant for each other. "Oh Ladybug, Honey, there is no way you can lose me. I'll be back five days after the furniture is in the house and the house is on the market."

"Honey, why can't you stay with me an extra day? I could call in sick and we would be together all day?"

"Ruth," I replied, "This is a trip I don't want to make to visit a lady I don't know. However, she has bought tickets to see 'Cats' because I told her to. It is only fair that I should be there at the time I said I would."

"Jay, I can't believe that you would still go and see that woman."

"Ladybug, I have to leave anyhow. I will get everything squared away in Santa Maria and return. That is a given. I will be coming back. But I did tell her I would be there, so I will keep my word. I will tell her about us meeting and that I intend to marry you. Since I have no attachment to her, I'm not sure it is really any of her business. But I intend to tell her in person, I think that is only right.

"These next seven days are not going to be fun, but I will be back in about two weeks. I will not be having sex with anything or anybody while I am gone."

I held her face between the palms of my hands and caressed her cheeks. "All I can say is that I love you. I want to stay, but I can't, there is a house to sell in Santa Maria. I will be back as soon as business is finished. Don't be angry with me, I can't stand the thought of you being mad or unhappy with me."

Ruth took my two hands in hers, and we stood there looking at each other. She smiled and said, "I'll bet the neighbors are watching and saying that this is better than television. I know that you have to go, so I guess I'll go to work. You might as well scram. Please drive safely, I do so want you back. Will you call me?"

I promised, "Every night until I get back. We are teenagers about four times over, and yet we act as if we are infected with puppy love. I know I am infected; all I am missing are the fleas."

Ruth laughed, and said, "Oh you, get going and get back here."

She whispered in my ear, "I miss you already", then she gave me a hard hug and a long kiss. I broke away, made a three hundred and sixty-degree turn while waving at the neighbors, got in the car, and drove away.

\*\*\*

My round trip, from Ypsilanti to Santa Maria and back again, was a joyless interlude that lasted far longer than I had planned. Although I was gone for only twenty days, being separated from Ruth made the time seem endless. There were fresh emotions that I hadn't felt in years surging through my body. The only thing that I could think of was Ruth. I was in a hurry to get everything arranged in California, notify my daughters about the sea change in my life, and get back to Michigan. However, I ran into prolems getting things done as quickly as I wanted.

When I arrived in Arizona, my visit was anticlimactic. The lady I stopped off to see really had been a friend of Virginia's before we got married. I don't believe that I had either seen her, or talked to her, more than twice in all of our thirty-seven years of marriage. As it turned out, she had much more important things on her mind besides my visit. One of her sons, from one of her marriages, had just walked out of the closet and announced to her that he was gay. She was having a difficult time coping with this news, so we were both glad to see the end of my visit. Ruth never said so, but I know that she was relieved when I left Arizona completely unscathed, unscarred, and untouched.

My frustrations began after I reached California. When I first got to Santa Maria I went to the real estate agency that I had used to rent our house while Virginia and I were in Massachusetts. They had the house keys, so I needed to see them just to get into the house. During the two and a half years of my absence, they had done a good job of screening and accepting tenants, monitoring the house, paying the bills, and keeping me informed of any necessary maintenance. Of course they got a commission in exchange for their work, but their hard work and their efficiency were well worth the price they charged. They had the last renters out of the house about two weeks before I arrived, and then they had the house cleaned, painted, with all the utilities turned on, awaiting my return.

After going through all the necessary paper work and back bills, I asked the woman I was dealing with if she would be interested in acting as my agent to sell the house.

She told me that she only handled rental property, but that she would put me in good hands. She took me over to the sales section and introduced me to their head salesperson, Debbie Trimble.

Ms. Trimble was a small, trim woman in her mid thirties. Her hair was short, and she was dressed in a dark blue, conservative business suit with a white blouse. She wore wire rim glasses that she would nervously twirl in her left hand when she wasn't wearing them.

I told Ms. Trimble about my meeting Ruth and changing my plans. I now wanted to put my house up for sale. She explained that real estate was selling very slowly in central California because the California economy wasn't doing well. Being a saleswoman, and therefore an optimist, she did think the house would sell, but that the price might not be as high as it would have been a year ago. She also said, after I asked, that showing the house furnished could help sell it. An empty home left its faults and shortcomings exposed while a furnished home looked friendlier. For some reason the condition of the furniture seemed to interest prospective buyers almost as much as the condition of the house. That made sense to me. I signed papers that Debbie, as my agent, would inspect the house, appraise it, and sell it on my behalf.

After finishing all the business, I got the keys from the real estate people and got into my house. I called the moving company and they told me that the truck carrying my furniture had broken down in the desert and that it would be delayed at least four days before it arrived in Santa Maria. I called Ruth with the bad news. We talked for a long time trying to figure out when I would be able to start my drive back to Michigan, but, of course, we didn't come to any conclusion. Nothing could be decided until the furniture truck arrived. I felt a little depressed and cranky after we hung up.

Then, in a grim mood that had nothing to do with them, I decided it was time to call each of my daughters and tell them about Ruth and me. For the last few days I had been trying to think of the best way to inform them of my plans. The news would be completely unexpected and it would come as a total surprise; there was no easy way of breaking the news.

Originally, Ruth hadn't been happy with the way I intended to tell my daughters about us. Her opinion was that a long distance phone call would be impersonal and upsetting to each girl, especially since the loss of their mother was still fresh. She said that she wouldn't blame my kids for thinking that I was crazy and that she was intruding into their lives. I didn't disagree with her but I didn't know how else to break my news to my daughters except by phone. Two daughters lived in different parts of North Carolina and one lived in Texas. The only other way to talk to each of them personally would be to fly to Texas and then to North Carolina. When I asked her if she had any better suggestions, she admitted that she didn't and we had dropped the subject.

This was at a time when I did not feel comfortable with my daughters and I had no idea of what had caused the strain among us. After Ginny's death, they didn't come together, share their grief, and get help from each other. They each turned inward and away from each other. Slights and hurts, real and imagined, past and present, were not discussed among them. Instead, grievances and feelings remained inside and became magnified and distorted in all three of them.

The girls moved apart from each other in an aura of bad will. Their feelings ranged from indifference to hostility. It was not the best of times for me or for my daughters. Virginia would have been very upset had she seen how our daughters were treating each other.

They were also drifting away from me, and that surprised me. After my own experiences as a child, I had tried to be a parent who was always available. Not only was their upbringing my responsibility, it was also a job that I thoroughly enjoyed. We went on a lot of adventures together. We visited the frigate "Old Ironsides", walked through bird sanctuaries in Sharon and Norfolk, toured Boston's North End, explored Cape Ann, and spent countless hours ocean watching. I thought that we all had grown up together, so I was pained when I realized we had grown so far apart.

After they got married they each went their own way. What interested me was that each daughter followed a different Christian religious path, and each daughter was dogmatic about her own religion. Dogmatic people are no fun and they make me wince. Dogmatic daughters not only make me wince they also make me hide.

They believed they were religious but I considered them fanatics. For me, a truly religious person, no matter what faith or denomination, is a joy. To be religious is to act compassionately and lovingly, comforting people without making any judgements about them or their problems. Keeping his, or her, own eternal soul pure and ready for meeting their maker in the hereafter is the primary concern of a religious person. I have met only a few people whom I honestly thought were really religious.

A fanatic has a different attitude than a religious person. He, or she, insists that they know what is right for humanity. To them the path to salvation is narrow, and only those who agree with their view can walk that path. They seem not to be as interested in helping people get through the problems of life as they are in warning them about what awaits them in the hereafter. Fanatics think that they are prophets. I think that they are dictators.

If my daughters want to believe, that is absolutely their right. If I want to question, that is absolutely my right. I did not question their beliefs but they certainly questioned my disbeliefs. They would not leave the subject of my lack of faith alone, each daughter tried to show me the light as she saw the light.

What disturbed me the most was that their religion didn't seem to offer them any relief or solace for their own problems. Almost every time I spoke with them they were either uptight, or unhappy, or not feeling well. Their religions didn't seem to send their spirits soaring.

Cynthia lived in San Antonio, Julie lived in Raleigh, and Elizabeth lived in Charlotte. Julie and Elizabeth were within driving distance of each other but neither of the girls ever called or visited the other. Since I lived a long distance away from all of them, I would call each of my daughters every week to find out how she was doing.

My conversations with them were rarely pleasant for me and mostly consisted of either their religion or their own bad feelings towards their sisters. I would tell them that I did not call to discuss their sisters with them and that they should talk to each other about their feelings;they should resolve their own differences. As a result, these phone calls were always difficult because I could not establish any common ground or rapport with my daughters. As a father it was painful not to be able to get them to stop squabbling. I loved them but I could not stand them.

None of my daughters had ever heard of Ruth. She and I had parted years before they were born. Mrs. O had seen Cynthia and Julie when they were babies and all three of the girls had heard Ginny and me talk about Mrs. O, but we referred to her only as a mutual friend. I had no idea what they would say, or how they would react, when I told them that I was going to re-marry. I was prepared to have some interesting conversations with my daughters.

As always, I called them in chronological order. Cynthia, my oldest, had been a freshman at Wheaton College when she interrupted her education and married her high school sweetheart while he was in the Air Force. She got her degree in history, from Maryland, after taking part time classes for many years. She finally earned it while they were stationed in England. Cynthia was home schooling her three children because she believed that public schools suffer from drug and discipline problems, and she also wanted to give them their religious training.

After her husband retired from the Air Force, they bought an ice skating rink in San Antonio. The strain of trying to keep an under funded business alive and running, after it had been mismanaged for years, was slowly wearing on both of them. They spent most of their waking hours fighting for their rink. They were under tremendous emotional and financial pressure and had little time for anything else.

Cynthia listened as I told her about Ruth and me. She did not interrupt, nor she did not ask any questions. When I finished, she did ask a few questions about Ruth and her three daughters. Then she said, "Dad, I guess you are not asking for my approval or my opinion. I assume that you are telling me for information only, which is fine. If you are happy than I am happy for you. I will be anxious to meet her. Tell Ruth that I wish the two of you all the happiness in the world." We talked about my immediate plans for a while and then I hung up. One down, two to go.

Julie, my middle daughter, had recently moved to Greensboro. Julie had a quick, hot temper and a fast tongue and sometimes she tried not to let reason interfere with her decisions. She first married right out of high school and was divorced a few years later. She graduated from High Point College and is quick to point out that her degree is in business. I always suspected that she got a strong minor in partying. She feels that she has never had a job equal to her capabilities and that she never had a boss as smart as she is and, as a result, she has a chip on her shoulder. Julie is not a happy person. Her second husband is an airplane mechanic and he is a placid, mild person. He provides a gentle balance for Julie and is a good father to their one child, a daughter. Julie had gone through the harrowing experience of having her mother die in bed, beside her, while she was pregnant. Then, she had to lie in the same bed three more months until her own child was born.

I expected problems with Julie when I called and told her about Ruth and me and my expectations were met and exceeded. She interrupted me before the first sentence was out of my mouth, and I could not finish any sentence without her asking two or three questions. Her questions were legitimate but the tone of the questions was offensive. Since it was her right to ask, I tried to answer every question quietly and patiently. She did not ask any questions about either Ruth or Ruth's daughters. Her questions dealt strictly with me. Did I feel all right? Was I depressed? Have I been having headaches lately? Was I losing my memory?

Since I knew that this news had to be a major shock for Julie I was as honest and as open as I could possibly be. When I had finished bringing her up to date on my plans, Julie said, "I don't approve of this, Daddy."

My own temper, which had been on edge, rose. I swallowed it and replied, "Julie, Honey, I did not call to get your approval. I called to tell you what I am planning on doing. I do not like telling you this over a telephone, I would have preferred seeing you face to face. Still, a phone call is better than not telling you at all. I was hoping that you would be happy for me, but I guess that isn't to be."

"No Dad, that isn't correct, I am happy for you, but this is so sudden I have to think. Let me get back to you in a few days." And with that, Julie hung up.

Well that takes care of two out of three, I thought.

Elizabeth, my youngest, lived in Charlotte, and she was the easiest daughter to talk with. She had always been a ray of sunshine in

Ginny's life until she married someone whom Ginny did not like. What bothered Ginny about Elizabeth's husband was not his personality; it was his religion. At the time Elizabeth married Brent, which was after she graduated from High Point College, he was a born again Christian. Ginny, a staunch and true Episcopalian, could not stand his views, and she made no secret of that fact. She railed against Elizabeth's husband and constantly scolded Elizabeth.

Elizabeth was caught in the middle between her husband and her mother, and her sunshine faded. She went from a loving daughter to a confused person trying to get her mother to accept her husband. The death of Ginny hurt Elizabeth because it left all of the tension between them unresolved. Elizabeth has been unsure of herself for years.

When I called Elizabeth and told her about Ruth and me, she almost cheered. She gushed with happiness over the phone and she made me repeat the story twice. She then wrote down Ruth's name and address and swore that she was going to write a note to her. I chuckled as I hung up because Elizabeth was the only one of my daughters who had taken the news in the way that I had hoped they all would.

I had spoken to the girls during the day. That evening, I called Ruth just after she arrived home from work. We had decided that was the best time to call, and I had spoken to her at least once a day since I left.

When I recounted the conversations, Ruth questioned me in detail about each girl's reaction. She wanted to know if I thought that their feelings had been hurt and if they were upset with her. I answered her questions, and she told me, again, that using a phone to pass on this kind of information was hard on the girls and that we had a lot of fence mending to do. Then we went on to other business.

Ruth asked, "Do you know where your furniture is?"

"Still on the truck, still in the desert, and still headed for Santa Maria," I replied. "They are supposed to give me a definite answer when I call their 800 number later on this evening. They will tell me where the truck is and when I can expect to see it in front of my house."

There was no reply. In fact, there was such a long pause that I finally asked, "Ruth?"

She spoke in a very small, soft voice, "Honey, this isn't just an excuse because you have changed your mind is it?"

I replied immediately, "Ladybug, I haven't changed my mind. It ain't my mind that has a problem, it is my heart. I miss you terribly.

"I will gladly give you the 800 number

and you can try your luck. If you can get them to deliver the furniture any faster than I can it wouldn't hurt my feelings.

"Have you changed your mind?"

Ruth replied vigorously, "Hell no, I haven't changed my mind. I consider us so lucky. But I do miss you and I am impatient for you to come back to me."

"I am impatient to get back," I said. "Here is what is going to happen while I am waiting for the furniture. The real estate agent will need me around for two or three more days. There are papers to sign and she wants to look at a couple of things in the house. Also, there is some furniture that was stored here in Santa Maria because the apartment back in Westboro was not as big as this house. That furniture will come out of storage and will be delivered tomorrow.

"Then, as soon as the furniture from Massachusetts is unloaded, I'm out of here. In the meantime, I just sit around without too much to do except constantly think of you."

Neither of us was happy during the next few days; they seemed to crawl by while we were separated from one another. However, the furniture truck finally did arrive, and all the arrangements to sell the house were completed. I was free to leave.

The day before my departure I got an angry letter from Julie. Without meeting Ruth or knowing anything about her Julie wrote that she did not think I should get married because she was concerned about my money after I died. She said that some of the money I now had was from her mother's estate and should go to her daughters. Julie felt that there was a chance that she would be cheated out of her inheritance.

She had leapfrogged way ahead of Ruth and me. Finance was the last thing on my mind. I had not thought about money and I doubted that Ruth had given it any thought either. We would have to get to it eventually, along with a host of other matters, but I was not concerned about Ruth. I was more concerned about Julie because I was not at all pleased with her letter and I intended to let her know about it.

My finances were absolutely none of Julie's business. I could have sympathized with Julie if she opposed Ruth because she did not like her, or if she thought Ruth's character was flawed. But to oppose my marriage because of her inheritance? That was absolute rubbish. Julie surprised me because she seemed out of character. Why the hell should Julie be counting my pennies?

I wrote her a letter back in which I told her that my finances were not her concern. When my death finally lifted the veil and revealed my estate, then it would be her business. Until that time, I felt free to use my money as I wished to use my money. I also told her I took her letter as a slap at Ruth and that was something I did not appreciate. I was going to marry Ruth and Julie would have to decide either to accept Ruth or to lose me. I was harsh in my response but I felt that her letter was way out of bounds.

That evening, I told Ruth about receiving a letter from Julie and I would let her read it when I got home. Ruth surprised me by telling me that she had gotten a nice note from Elizabeth saying she was glad to hear the news of our plans. So, the score was tied and Cynthia was the tiebreaker. I said to Ruth that she shouldn't be concerned, all three girls would not only accept her, they would quickly learn to love her.

She was skeptical. I wasn't. Although my daughters and I didn't agree on much, I knew what their basic values were. After all, I had helped instill them. Once they met Ruth, they would succumb to her warmth, honesty, and charm exactly as their father had done.

The next morning, I started my return trip back to Michigan. I drove over the speed limit, I drove long hours, I stopped only to rest or relieve myself. I was in an absolute fury to get back. When I reached Ypsilanti, I moved in with Ruth and, without benefit of clergy, we started to live together as husband and wife.

It had only taken me slightly more than forty years to get my act together.

***

Living together was easy. Despite the forty years that had intervened, we were still deeply in love. It was a legal narcotic that we delightfully gave, ardently took, and our supply never diminished. We shared our laughs, tears, angers, hurts, and joys.

The difference, between the first time we met and this time, was our maturity. My present emotions, which had lain dormant like a sleeping volcano, were just as passionate as they were when I was young, but time had taught me how to handle the molten feelings. I was no longer hiding from myself or deferring to others. What you saw from me was absolutely what you got, warts and all. Take it or leave it. Ruth was also direct, straightforward and candid but, undoubtedly, she was much more diplomatic than I was. The result was a union that was joyous. It was honest, strong, and respectful. And, best of all, it could be prickly at times.

When we had decisions, or choices, to make we would make ourselves comfortable and review our options. We would defer to each other when we could, or simply agree to disagree when we could not. A few times our exchanges were heated; but neither of us walked away wearing a fake smile that hid a masked anger. We had too much faith in each other to harbor resentments, we both knew that life was short.

We did not just live together, we were partners. We came to each other with differences in personalities, ideas, attitudes and sex. Even though we were both strong willed, we made it work because we wanted it to work. Our rekindled love gave us a passion for life and living was a marvelous experience. We would never give up on each other again; we were well matched and truly united.

However, even Heaven must have some kind of organization and, to begin with, we were in complete disarray. Ruth had lived alone for many years and the house was filled and cluttered to her satisfaction. There was absolutely no room for me; it even took a few weeks for Ruth to find one single drawer for me to put away my socks and underwear. Now that we were together, we each had to make changes in what had been our individual life styles, especially since Ruth worked and I did not.

My status was that I had been laid off, and, as soon as my layoff benefits ran out, I would retire. So, I was staying at home and Ruth was going to work and she wanted to keep working.

Ruth's initial concerns were not so much about our living arrangements as they were about her daughters and me. She wanted her daughters to get to know, and love me. When I returned from California she immediately addressed this situation because she was not at all sure how they were going to react to her having a man in her life.

As it turned out, Ruth's three girls were much more receptive about our relationship than my girls had been. Both sets of daughters were protective of their parents, but both had had entirely different upbringings. Ruth's girls had been raised in Ypsilanti, and the house that Ruth lived in was the only home they had ever known. When they were very young their father went from a practicing dentist to a philandering drunk whose license was revoked. They saw their home life as a constant series of fights that had left their mother upset and angry. As they grew up, went to high school, got married, and left home, they were witnesses to the struggles their mother went through to raise them and provide what she could.

One of Ruth's biggest disappointments was that none of her daughters had gone to college. She even had a hard time getting them through high school. Despite the fact that she wanted them to continue their education, they did not listen to her. She told them that she would manage to raise the money for their education. I guess she would have borrowed money from her mother and father if it had become necessary. She wanted them to go to college and do what she had not done, live on campus. She felt that going to school and living in a dorm would broaden their horizons, equip them to earn a better living and give them a feel for some of the finer things in life. Because her daughters got jobs after high school instead of going to college, she was unhappy and she blamed herself.

Like most offspring, her daughters did not appreciate or understand the struggles their mother went through until they themselves married and began to raise families. Then, as if to make amends for the problems they had caused her, her daughters never strayed far from Ruth.

And her dedication to them had been total. After the hurt and bitterness of her marriage faded, she never got involved with another man. She was not sure how her daughters would be accepted, or treated, by any of the men she met and dated and her daughters were her first responsibility. She stood aloof from any emotional involvement. Even after I returned, she was defensive of her daughters and her grandchildren until she realized that I treated her tribe the same way that I treated my own.

It is true that many second marriages have problems because of the children of either spouse. It's difficult not to want to protect your own and think the worst of the others. That was a trap that both Ruth and I were able to avoid. We tried to be honest enough to judge both sets of girls by the same standards, and our children never became an issue. Between us, we had six daughters who could be annoying, aggravating, pleasing, or whatever other emotion daughters evoke; but we did have six daughters, not three of hers and three of mine.

It was easier, and more personal, to notify her daughters of our intentions than it was to notify my daughters. We did it together and in person. Her three daughters came over to the house, one at a time, with their spouses, or, in her oldest daughter's case, with her live-in boy-friend, to meet me. Like my daughters, who had never heard of Ruth, her daughters had never heard of me. They each met me, spent time visit-ing, and then left. Since their mother was now happier than they had ever before seen her, they were eager to accept me. Of course, when each girl got home she immediately called the other two, compared notes, and then each girl called Ruth and told her what all three had to say. I couldn't help but notice that Ruth's daughters talked continually together. I don't believe my daughters even bothered to call each other after I told them about Ruth and me. I wished they had.

Robin, Ruth's oldest, is an attractive, intelligent girl who bore the brunt of the terrible times of her mother's failed marriage. She is the only daughter not presently married although she does have a son from a previous marriage. After her mother's divorce, while she was still a young teenager, her father tried to sexually assault her. Growing up, she was wild and hard to manage. She has difficulty making up her mind, and prefers that others make her decisions for her. Ruth always felt that, if Robin had gone to college, she could have accomplished anything she wanted; I think Ruth was right.

Christie, the middle daughter, is a chatterbox and is delightful to have around. She is enthusiastic, upbeat, and sweet. Tracy and Robin look to Christie for advice because she is dependable. But she also can be unpredictable. She works at The Michigan Secretary of State's office and efficiently handles problems with car registrations, driver's licenses, and automobile insurance. However, she manages to lose her own car keys almost every time she gets out of her car. She makes me laugh because her conversations seem scatterbrained; however, when she faces a problem, her decisions are mature and wise.

Tracy is Ruth's youngest daughter. Ruth and her sisters were overly protective of Tracy; they have always thought of her as the baby of the family. She grew up as a very headstrong person who did whatever she wanted whenever she wanted. At night, she would hot wire Ruth's car while Ruth was sleeping for midnight joy rides. She isn't the slightest bit mean, just bull-headed. When Tracy had her own two daughters she realized how much grief she had caused Ruth, and, ever since, she has tried to make amends for her childhood behavior.

The three of Ruth's girls are closer together, as friends and sisters, than the three of my girls. Ruth's girls cling to their mother, and to each other, in order to keep their family ties intact. Despite their different personalities and differences of opinions, they are linked with one another, as sisters, for the rest of their lives. I wish my girls had adopted that same attitude. It is much more than distance that separates my daughters. I guess they each feel too hurt to forget the past and start over.

The first discussions between Ruth and me, concerning our living together, were about how we were going to pay our normal living expenses. I told Ruth that the answer was simple. She had a checking account while I didn't, I had closed mine when I left Massachusetts. And, since I was drawing a paycheck every two weeks until my layoff benefits ran out, I would deposit my check in her checking account. She would add my name to the account and then we could each write checks to take care of our expenses.

She thought that was a good idea until I told her how big my paycheck was. She protested that my paycheck was much bigger than her paycheck and that the arrangement would not be equitable. I replied that I did not consider it as her money or my money. It was money for each of us to spend however we wished. It took a while before Ruth got used to having a large checking account, but it also took a much longer time for her to buy whatever she wanted whenever she wanted.

In the past, her financial advisor had told her that if she planned on traveling after retiring, she would have to work way past the normal retirement age. She conceded that now there was enough money for us to enjoy a good life style and to travel anywhere in the world if we wanted. However, she enjoyed working and she wanted to keep her independence. She had been independent for years and her independence was important to her. So, she decided to continue working. I did not agree with her decision, but I did not argue. I valued my own independence too much to interfere with hers.

Her work dictated the rhythm of our daily lives. During the week, when we didn't eat out, I would prepare the meals. I enjoyed cooking and that made life easier for Ruth. I would also do as much housecleaning and yard work, as Ruth would allow. However, there were certain chores that she would not let anyone do for her. She insisted on keeping the laundering, ironing, and the planting of flowers as jobs that were her responsibility.

We had only one bathroom and that was a problem, a big problem. I would try to stay clear of it while she readied herself for work. That sometimes proved to be difficult because Ruth was very particular about her appearance. She would fuss over colors and dawdle over earrings, forgetting that she was not by herself any more, while, on the other hand, I would be dancing a jig and almost wetting my pants. There has to be a lot of love and compassion between a man and a woman to stay together while sharing only one toilet.

There was one thing that I insisted on immediately changing. I went out, bought a coffeepot and freshly ground coffee and replaced the instant coffee that we had in the morning. The

smell of brewing coffee, and the taste of freshly made coffee, helped both of our dispositions
while Ruth got ready for work in the mornings.

Although I was not working I was rarely
idle. I would get phone calls from my friends
and my former coworkers from Vandenberg,
Hill, and Norton Air Force Bases and from Boston and Seattle. At first, the calls were a mix of
personal and professional questions. I enjoyed
talking shop about the Minuteman Missile. My
opinion was occasionally solicited on a few system changes that I had been working on. I had
worked on Minuteman for almost twenty-five
years and I was familiar with how it operated.
Soon though, the professional calls tapered off
and I was out of the technical loop. All of my
phone calls, from then on, were personal.

My main occupation, though, was preparing to go from layoff status into retirement. Sorting out the paperwork to understand the transition was almost a full time job. Transferring
thirty years of retirement funds, stock options,
employee stock option plans, and health benefits from GTE's control to my own, while staying within the Internal Revenue Service rules,
was complicated. And changing these accounts
to maintain my own best interests was also difficult. What made all of this work so confusing
was the fact that all of my business was done

over the phone. I would get one answer, from someone, to a question one day, and the next day the same question would bring an entirely different response from a different person.

Adding to the confusion of all of this was the fact that when I became eligible for Social Security in less than a year, some of my insurance benefits and my retirement options would be changed. It took me a long time to read all the brochures and documents and a lot of phone calls to finally understand what I was doing. Because I was only going to be able to do this once, I needed to get it right. Going over each and every detail time after time was no fun, and I swore a lot, but I knew the importance of doing it correctly.

***

As Ruth and I became more intimate with each other, our individual personalities began to mesh more closely. We each had an inherent desire to please our partner and to share our joy with each other. As a result, we made up words, phrases, and rituals that we meant only for our own use. We did not go out of our way to invent them, rather they seemed to happen and flow between us easily and naturally. Doing them gave us the pleasure of togetherness. They were small things but they were personal and important parts of our lives and we treasured them. They became the steel rebars that prevented the concrete of our alliance from developing cracks.

It all began with endearments. Ruth almost always called me, "Honey." I began by calling her "Ladybug" and that is what I usually called her. Soon though, I alternated that with "PITA", Pain In The Ass. After we were married, I also called her "Wife", but I purposely mispronounced it as whiff.

One ritual started when we came home from some friends of ours after a night of drinking. It was about two in the morning and we were both tired and a little drunk. When we pulled into the driveway, I turned the motor off and I said, "Home again, home again jiggety jig."

Ruth asked, "What was that?"

"That's from the nursery rhyme,
To market, to market,
To buy a fat pig,
Home again, home again, jiggety jig."

The next few times we came home late, I repeated the last line each time I shut off the motor. Just after I said that, one time in particular, Ruth responded by saying, "Home again, home again jiggety jog."

I asked her, "What was that?"

She said, "Hah, how soon they forget.

That's the second verse,
> To market, to market,
> To buy a fat hog,
> Home again, home again, jiggety jog"

After a while, we cut it down to my saying, "Jiggety jig," and Ruth replying, "Jiggety jog." After a long day, or a late night, we never got out of the car without each of us saying our part.

Eating in a restaurant one night we began one of the few rituals that we did both in public and when we were alone at home. Generally, we ate out almost every weekend. After being served a before dinner drink, I was raising mine to take a drink when Ruth glared at me and asked, "Excuse me, but aren't we going to make a toast?"

I quickly put the drink back on the table and said. "Oops, my mistake. Sure we should make a toast. Why don't you make it?"

She smiled at me, we touched our glasses together, and she said, "Klunk, I love you, Jay."

I replied, "Klunk, I love you, Ruth."

From that time on, we always klunked to each other before our first drink. When I made an occasional mistake, and forgot to klunk with her, Ruth let me know about my gaffe in no uncertain terms.

The ritual that we both cherished the most came about because I generally woke up earlier than Ruth and I enjoyed lying there, watching her as she slept. Her face was careworn, she had certainly gone through a lot during her lifetime, but that only added to her beauty. At first, Ruth was nonplussed when she would wake up and find me looking at her. Then, she decided to take advantage of this chance for verbal sparring.

Ruth might ask, "Are you getting your money's worth?"

I would reply, "I haven't made up my mind yet. Why?"

"Before you do, Buster, there is something you should know. Nothing in this world is free, so because you have been peeking, leave an extra ten bucks on the bureau when you decide to leave."

Or, she might ask, "What are you looking at?"

"I am just trying to figure out which one of us is the prettiest," I would reply.

She would smile and answer, "Listen, if you are interrupting your sleep just for that, you must really be worried."

Or, she might say, "Oh my God, there is a naked man in my bed."

"Ladybug, don't hand me that line, you are the one that seduced me."

"Now that is absolutely not true, because I am not that type of girl. There must have been drugs involved."

From then on, after our opening ploys, we would snuggle for a few minutes and talk over our individual schedules and what had to be done that day. Our love huddles were fairly short during weekdays, because Ruth had to work, but they were an important start to our days. On weekends, they were long and leisurely. We eventually gave them the name of coo and cluck sessions.

One morning Ruth started our coo and cluck session by saying, "Jay, I really should hate you."

"Any particular reason for this outburst, or is it just a generic thing?" I asked.

"Oh yes, there is a specific reason," Ruth replied. "Did you know, that after almost every letter that my mother received from you, she would tell me, 'Jay has a good job. You should have married him.'"

I looked directly at Ruth, and said, "Lady-bug, this is the very first time I heard that. Of course I didn't know. That was terrible. Awful. I wouldn't have blamed you if you had been angry. No, I knew nothing about it. Why would she do such a thing?"

"I don't know," Ruth said. "I often wondered why you two were even writing to each other. You told me that she never mentioned me in her letters?"

"That's what I said, not at all. Never once did she mention you. I didn't know you were divorced, I didn't know you lived in Ypsi, I didn't know anything about you until I got the letter that she asked you to write to me."

She looked at me, and asked seriously, "Honey, do you think that she was always thinking of us getting together again?"

"I don't know, Ruth. I wasn't such a good prospect forty years ago. Maybe the possibility was always in the back of her mind. She certainly gave me no hint of that, although I often wondered why she kept in touch. I am glad that she did."

"Me too, Honey. I am so glad that you came back to visit my mother."

There was nothing more meaningful for either of us than being able to relax, hold our partner, and share our thoughts and feelings. Our coo and cluck sessions bared our weaknesses and our frailties to each other. We each confessed our fears and our frights, and in so doing, we became more entwined. The force field that surrounded Ruth and me, which started as an attraction so many years ago, was as invisible and invincible as gravity. Life was sweet to us and we were happy.

Sunday mornings became a ritual in themselves. We were usually up by 6:30AM and, because Ruth didn't have to go work and we had no errands to run, we would try to make time pass in slow motion. A long coo and cluck session was followed by a leisurely cup of coffee and then we would turn our attention to the New York Times Sunday crossword puzzle in the Detroit News. Ruth would always make the entries because her handwriting was so much better than my scribbling. In making the entries, she displayed the one affectation that I ever saw from her. She would never use a pencil to write the answers, instead, she would always use a ballpoint pen. She not only had confidence in her ability to solve crossword puzzles she wanted everyone to know that she was confident. She was proud of her ability to do crosswords. The downside of this was that, when a mistake was made, the correction was messy.

We would sit side by side at the dinette table. The room was dark and the ceiling fixture did not cast enough light on the table. We would turn on two floor lamps but we still had reading difficulties. The print was small and we had occasional problems making out the words. Despite these minor inconveniences, we looked forward to doing the crossword puzzle together. Once or twice, the paper was delivered late and Ruth was annoyed that our routine was delayed.

We would work without using a dictionary or any references. Since she was the one who wielded the pen, Ruth made the final decisions. Usually, we would finish the puzzle in an hour or two. Sometimes it would take two to three hours to finish, and, when it took that long, we would look up the troublesome words in whatever reference we had on hand. When we did encounter definitions we couldn't solve, we would buy the Detroit News on Monday to see the answers to the words that had baffled us. Between the two of us, it was a rarity when we couldn't complete the crossword puzzle.

Of course it was not all sweetness. Both Ruth and I were much too salty and purposeful to feel that we had to agree to get along. We had some very sturdy disagreements, and we both relished them. Sometimes Ruth was right, sometimes I was right, sometimes we were both wrong. It didn't matter who was right or who was wrong, we had nothing to prove to one another so we could disagree, agree to disagree, laugh about it, and get on with enjoying each other.

Our coo and cluck sessions taught me something profound. I used to think that love was like the mathematical term infinity; so huge that it is boundless. Our love transcended that.

It made infinity as tiny as a grain of sand lying on a bowling alley.

***

Prior to my return, Ruth had been visiting her mother twice a week. She would go to the nursing home every Wednesday evening straight from work, and then, whenever she had free time, on either Saturday or Sunday. These were dutiful, rather than joyful, visits because talking to her mother was difficult.

Also, Ruth couldn't forget that her mother had never lavished any affection on her. As a mother, Mrs. O was cold and aloof. Ruth told me that, a few years before he died, her father had told her that it was on his wedding night when he learned that he had made a mistake. She said that her father did not elaborate but that she had known what he meant. Ruth always wondered if her mother had ever engaged in sex more than the two times it was necessary for both of her children to be conceived.

Growing up was an unhappy experience for both Ruth and her brother, Edward. Edward got out of the house, by joining the navy as soon as he was of age, and he never came back. Mrs. O had always told Ruth that, while she was pregnant with Ruth, she had wanted another boy and not a daughter. Yet, in spite of all her unpleasant memories, Ruth felt that she was obligated to make her mother's life as pleasant as possible.

Since Ruth was working, I volunteered to take over the Wednesday visits to ease her load and then we could both go together during the weekend. At first, Ruth protested about me going alone on Wednesday. She knew that visiting her mother was difficult, and she felt that it was her responsibility, not mine, to make these visits. I agreed with her that it was difficult, but I disagreed with her that it was her responsibility alone. I considered both of us as a unit, and as such, Ruth could not divide our responsibilities just by herself. Both of us talking together was the way I wanted to face problems and work out solutions. Finally, after a lot of discussion, Ruth reluctantly agreed to let me try a few visits by myself.

After I had made two or three of the Wednesday visits alone, Ruth began to realize that her mother didn't care whether or not Ruth came along. Mrs. O was just grateful to have anyone interrupt her long days and nights of lying in bed. She lay there, unable to see or hear well, her mind trapped inside the prison of her deteriorating body. Ruth admitted that my weekday visits made her life easier and she didn't have any guilty feelings that her mother was being neglected. She didn't change her mind about it being her responsibility to go see her mother but she did stop objecting to my going by myself.

And visiting her mother was a chore, a sad chore. No matter what Mrs. O's faults had been when Ruth was growing up, this once proud, fierce, woman was now reduced to being a frail skeleton with her muscles hanging off her bones. She was in her eighties and her active mind was beginning to fail, hidden from our view on the other side of partial blindness and partial deafness. What were her thoughts during those long hours and days between visits? How did she occupy her time? I often wondered.

Each of my visits began with a check of her bedside flowers. If her carnations had been droopy on the last visit, I would bring a new bouquet on my next visit; if they were still fresh, I would trim their stems and change the water. She was always given red carnations because she could see red easier than white or pink. I would hold them close to her so that she could try to count them and then smell them.

After the flowers were placed on her bedside table, I would sit near her and try to hold a conversation. Occasionally, she would be alert and receptive and talking would be enjoyable.

Most of the time, though, she was not responsive and I would have to repeat myself often and loudly for her to hear. I am sure that our conversations echoed down the entire length of the nursing home hall.

While trying to talk, I would offer her fruit and candy. Her favorite fruit was fresh raspberries, but when I couldn't buy them, she never turned down pieces of cantaloupe. She had to be hand fed with a spoon, one small piece of fruit at a time, and that was a slow, messy procedure.

After she finished the fruit, I would offer her a piece of soft centered candy from a box of chocolates we kept in her room closet. She would hold the candy in her trembling hand and nibble. By the time she finished, her fingers would be covered with melted chocolate and I would have to take a damp facecloth and wipe her hands and her face.

Near the end of the visit, which could last from one to three hours, I would offer to make Mrs. O a gin and tonic. Ruth had convinced her mother's doctor that it would be good for her to be allowed a drink whenever she had a visitor. So Mrs. O's private supplies were kept under lock and key, available for either Ruth or me when we wished to mix her a drink. I would fix a weak gin and tonic in a paper cup and hold it up to her when she was ready. She would suck it up a straw greedily, and one would usually put her right to sleep.

Although Mrs. O had played tennis when she was a girl, she had grown totally indifferent to sports, with one exception. She had always been a rabid Michigan football fan. When I was dating Ruth, it used to tickle me to see such a sophisticated woman rant and rave and swear at her radio when Michigan's opponents scored a touchdown. Now, during the football season, Ruth would call the nursing home on Saturday mornings and remind them to turn on either Mrs. O bedside radio or her television set so that her mother could follow the game. Even lying comatose for most of the time, Mrs. O would still root for her boys.

And she could still be feisty as hell. One Wednesday afternoon I came into her room, stood at the foot of her bed, watched her lying there with her eyes shut, and, for no particular reason at all, I said, "Good afternoon, Kathleen."

Her eyes opened immediately, she raised her head a little, and with absolutely no nonsense in the tone of her voice, she said, "I certainly have never given you permission to address me as Kathleen."

Mrs. O was extremely happy that I had returned and that Ruth and I were living together.

She had never liked Ruth's husband and she had been concerned for her daughter during the time Ruth was working and raising her family. When I came back, Mrs. O felt much easier about Ruth's future, but she wanted us to have a different relationship. She kept asking us "How soon before you two are going to get married?"

She told Ruth's daughters, "I just love that man." I laughed when they repeated the conversation to me and I said that, when Ruth and I were first going together, she did not feel quite that same way. It was only after I had left the scene that I began to look pretty good to her.

\*\*\*

Almost a year and a half would pass before Ruth finally met each of my daughters in person. There was no lack of communications during this time as I still called them once a week and Ruth usually talked on the phone as much as I did, if not longer. There were occasional letters exchanged from them to her; sometimes Ruth shared their contents with me before she replied, sometimes she replied without telling me what the subject was. When I returned to Ypsilanti we had talked about when we would travel to Texas and North Carolina to meet them. My daughters rarely took trips and we were busy establishing our new lives. I used to jokingly tell Ruth that her daughters lived much too close to us while mine lived much too far away. It was a family tragedy that brought about the first meeting between Ruth and one of my daughters.

We had been living together for less than three months, when, on the fourteenth of September, Cynthia called me. She was frantic and beside herself with grief. Her two-year old daughter, Jessica, her youngest child, had drowned in the family swimming pool. She, Allen, and their three other children, Courtney, Sarah, and Nicholas, were devastated. One minute, it was a family lark; the next minute, death had split the family.

I told Cynthia I would make travel plans to fly to San Antonio. When I hung up and broke the news to Ruth about Jessica's death, she cried. I called the airlines to find out about their schedules and their departure times but I did not make any reservations. Ruth and I had to decide whether she could, or should, come to San Antonio with me and, after that, I had to find out if Cynthia would be comfortable if Ruth did accompany me.

We had tickets that evening for a performance, in Detroit, of the music of Andrew Lloyd Webber. Ruth asked whether we should go to the concert or stay home. Rightly or wrongly, I figured that we would be better off continuing with our activities, so, I decided that we should go. We were both all right until the lights went down and the music began. Then the enormity of the personal tragedy hit us. We sat there, in the dark, listening to that beautiful music, tightly holding each other's hand, while tears streamed down our faces.

That night, when we were cuddled in bed, Ruth said, "Honey, I want to be with you in San Antonio. It is my place to be with you; but I do not how Cynthia would feel about my being there. After all, her mother died, and then you came to live with me, a total stranger whom she knew nothing about. Now she has this tragedy. The pain she has must be unimaginable. She has gone through enough. You will have to tell me what I should do, I don't want to cause her any more grief."

I said, "Ladybug, you could stay home. This isn't your problem."

Ruth's temper immediately flared. She said angrily, "Not my problem? What kind of bullshit is this? You give me this lecture about unity for both of us, about all of our problems being mutual, but I can't help you? What do we have here a double standard?"

Despite her anger, I had to laugh. "All right, all right, you are correct. I was just trying to save you from what is going to be a horrible time. I want you with me. When I talk to Cynthia, in the morning, I will ask her if she has any objections to your being with me."

Cynthia, with all of her other sorrows, raised no objections. Ruth and I flew to San Antonio for Jessica's funeral. Those four days were a time that I wish I could put behind me, but I will always remember them. Allen's brothers and sisters and mother were at the funeral. They are a rowdy, noisy, drinking family and they are damn good people to have around in bad times. Cynthia's three children were pathetic little bundles of pain. All three of them were abnormally quiet and still. They were constantly being handed over, from one adult to another to be hugged, kissed, and told to be brave.

When Ruth and I attended the funeral, we held hands even tighter than we did the night of the concert. I know that it was larger than it appeared, but that tiny white casket looked no bigger than a shoebox. I could not keep my eyes from it. I stared at it thinking of all the hurt, guilt, horror, shame, and sorrow that must be wrenching each member of Cynthia's family. Pain poured over us like acid rain and we were forever etched.

The night before we left, when Ruth and I were lying in bed, she asked, "Jay, do you know any of the details about Jessica's death?"

"No."

"Are you going to ask?" Ruth inquired.

"No."

"Why not? That's not like you, Jay. You usually try to find out everything."

"Ladybug, I am not sure that I really want to know, and I am not even sure it is important now. Everyone seems to be tiptoeing around the details. If anyone in the family made a mistake, or didn't pay attention, or just plain screwed up, what difference does it make now? Each member of this family is going through their own hell. I suspect something, but I don't know what, and they are reluctant to say much to me. So, I think I should let it go. What do you think?"

"I guess you are right, Honey. They will feel this for the rest of their lives." She paused a moment and then added, "Cynthia certainly is a big girl, just like Tracy."

"They both certainly are." I lay there for a moment, and then I kissed Ruth on the top of her head. "Ladybug, thank you for coming with me and helping me. I love you."

Ruth snuggled closer. She said, "I just wish there was more that I could do. I wish I could help Cynthia's pain. I wish I could help Cynthia and Tracy lose weight. I wish I could do more than I have done."

After a few moments of silence, Ruth asked, "What time does our plane leave in the morning?"

"It leaves about nine. We should be ready to leave the house by about seven."

Ruth said, "I sure will be glad to get home to our own bed. Do you think anyone can hear us in this bedroom?"

"I don't think so, Ruth. Allen's family is staying in a motel and this is the only bedroom on the first floor. All the other bedrooms are over another wing of the house on the second floor."

Ruth came much closer to me. "Don't ask me why, Jay, but suddenly I feel horny. Honey, do you think it would be terrible to do it right here, right now?"

I certainly did not, and we certainly did.

The next morning we said goodbye and flew back to Michigan.

The emotional battering we suffered on the trip to San Antonio may have contributed to the delay before Ruth met Julie and Elizabeth. It was not until after we were married that we took a trip to the Outer Banks of North Carolina and, during the trip, we stopped in to meet them. We visited Elizabeth in Charlotte and Julie in Greenville. Elizabeth was delighted to meet Ruth and Julie, who had gotten over her pique long ago, was also pleased. For her part,

Ruth had no reservations about her feelings for my daughters.

***

Two months after we returned from San Antonio, we went out to celebrate the fifth month anniversary of our reunion. We had just been served our first round of drinks, a screwdriver for me, and a gin and tonic for Ruth. We touched glasses, both of us said, "Klunk, I love you," and smiled at each other.

"Ruth," I said, "I really hate to bother you but I have to know whether you intend to make an honest man of me or not."

"Honey, what is the hurry? Do you have another offer?"

"No," I replied. "Not this week, anyhow. But I have been meaning to ask you if your intentions are honorable."

"Oh Jay, Honey, they always are. We will get married, but I don't know exactly when. Does that bother you?"

I chuckled and answered, "No, Ladybug, it doesn't bother me in the slightest. As a matter of fact, I rather enjoy it. I really don't give a damn, as long as we are together. Your mother keeps asking me about our marriage, when she thinks about it, and my own daughters ask occasionally. Living with you is fun, living with you in sin, is spicy fun. I am satisfied."

When we had finished our meal, and were lingering over coffee, Ruth reached across the table and patted my hand. She said, "Honey, I know you think that I can never make up my mind about anything, but that is not what is holding me back. I do love you. I have never felt as secure and happy as I now do. I just don't like changes. I had a bad experience once, and I am so happy now that I am almost afraid to change. If you are unhappy about our living together we can get married anytime. There really is no reason not to get married."

"Listen, Ladybug, we won't get married until you are either in a family way, or you decide it is time to get married. What is important to me is that we are together."

After that evening, because Ruth had taken my bantering so seriously, I decided not to say another word about marriage. Unless Ruth brought the subject up, I was not interested. And that was the way it remained, until I got a package from GTE.

I was listed on their roster as laid off. By their definition, I was still an active employee and could be recalled to work, although that was most unlikely. I would be listed as laid off until my banked vacation time and my accrued lay off time expired. After that period, which was due to last another six months, I would retire. Technically, since I wasn't retired, I was an active employee.

The information I received was an attempt to speed up the retirement of all active employees by offering a sweetened retirement package. I studied the material for a day and then I made several phone calls to the GTE Human Resources office to make sure that I had correctly interpreted the new information they sent to me. When I had finished deliberating, it was time to talk to Ruth; we had decisions to make.

When Ruth got home from work, she went to freshen up and change clothes, while I mixed us both a drink. We "klunked", and instead of letting the conversation drift I steered it.

"Listen Ruth," I began, "I have finished going through that package of information that I got from GTE two days ago. It is a carrot that they are dangling in front of us older donkeys because they want us to get the hell off the road. And, as a retirement package, it is a little sweeter than I would get if I waited for my normal retirement."

"Jay, Honey, I am much too old to believe in either Santa Claus or The Tooth Fairy. There must be a catch in this, somewhere."

"Well there is, Ladybug. And this is where

you are going to be rubbed the wrong way. But let me finish with what I was telling you first. The carrot is that I add about twenty thousand dollars to my lump sum retirement, and that money can be rolled over to my retirement account. Also, if I take this retirement package, and you and I are married before I retire, you will be covered by my medical insurance, and GTE will pay for ninety percent of the cost of both of our health insurance premiums."

Ruth sat there thinking about what I had told her. She mulled this information over before she said anything. Finally, she asked, in a very cold tone, "And what if you and I are not married by the time this elegant package takes effect?"

"If we are not married at the time I retire, I will get single medical coverage and they pay ninety percent of the premium. When we do marry, I can get you covered by the insurance, but we will have to pay one hundred percent of your premium."

Ruth flared up, "God Damn it. Son of a bitch. Some bean counter in GTE is trying to force me into marriage. That is just plain bullshit."

I sat quietly for a few seconds until she calmed down. "No, Ruth, I promise you that no one is going to force you into anything. I have told you this before, if you don't feel ready to get married we will not get married."

Ruth stopped being angry. "Honey, it has nothing to do with being ready." She smiled, "It is not really such a chore for me to marry you. I just feel that I am being pushed. You know that I am too tight to spend an extra couple of thousand dollars a year on premiums if I don't have to. It is just that I wanted to make up my own mind, not have some damn electronic company do it for me."

She reached over and touched my arm. "I guess that sounds ungracious of me and I don't mean it to be. If it is good for you, than it is good for us. How much time does GTE give us before this shotgun wedding has to take place?"

"All of our paperwork has to be completed, and in their hands in about two weeks."

Ruth got angry again. "Son of a bitch, what a bunch of assholes. Why can't they give us a decent time to decide? I hate them. Is there anything else that you have to tell me?"

"No, Ladybug, you now know as much as I do. Honey, in one sense it doesn't make much difference. If we don't take this package now, the same insurance problem will come up whenever I do retire. If we are not married, we will have to pay for your premium ourselves."

Ruth did not say a word. I knew that she

was angry and I also knew she was thinking over what I had said. That evening she called each of her daughters. That was a bit unusual because, recently, she had not been bothering to call unless she had not heard from them in a few days. She had been content to loosen their reins a little. I did not hear the conversations, but from the tone of her voice, I knew she was not happy.

After we were in bed and snuggling, Ruth said, "Honey, I hope that I have not hurt your feelings. I do love you. I will walk down the aisle and marry you willingly, gladly, and with all my heart. I just hate to be told that I have to by a group of executives who are high priced bean counters and who have little regard for human emotions."

"Ruth, I understand. I have no doubt about what you feel for me. We probably will marry sooner or later. It really does not matter to me because, right now, I am content. If you are not ready, we won't take this package. The money means nothing to me if you are not comfortable. If you have any questions or doubts, don't do it. Husband and wife, lovers, significant others, the names don't mean a damn thing to me. We are together and that is all I really care about."

Ruth sighed, moved closer, and replied, "Sweetie, I hate to make decisions but I have never been able to pass up a bargain. Could we get all the paperwork ready in time for the deadline?"

"I think so, but I am not sure. We will have to find a state that does not require either blood tests or a two-week waiting period before issuing a license. I could look that up in the Ypsilanti library tomorrow morning. But what about Mimi and Tom?"

Mimi had been Ruth's best friend from the time they met and they had known each other since they were teenagers. Ruth had been the bridesmaid at Mimi and Tom's wedding but Mimi hadn't been the bridesmaid at Ruth's wedding. When Ruth got married, Mimi and Tom were living in California and could not get to Ann Arbor. Ruth had often told me that she wanted Mimi as her bridesmaid when we got married.

"Damn it, Jay, this is all so complicated. What are we going to do?"

I smiled. Although Ruth didn't like to make decisions, I knew that she was going to have to quickly make up her mind. She really was in a quandary. I rubbed her fanny, more for solace than sex. "Well, we surely are not going to come to any conclusions right now. Let's see what we find out tomorrow."

By mid-morning of the next day, I began to see that the pieces of our wedding puzzle could be put together. A trip to the library, and a Xerox machine, gave me a list of marriage requirements for each state. Ruth immediately ruled out Michigan as a possible marriage site because of family considerations. If we were married in Michigan, and Michigan did meet our requirements, her three daughters would absolutely make it to our wedding, but my daughters would either be left out, or have to spend a lot of money to get here. By getting married somewhere else, none of our six daughters would be able to afford the travel and motel expenses. There would be peace at no financial cost to any family member.

Ruth looked at the list and noticed that we could get married in Nevada. She said that she would like to be married in Lake Tahoe because the scenery was beautiful and it was close to where Mimi and Tom lived. So, we decided to get married in Nevada.

After we started talking and making plans Ruth began to get excited. She reminded me that I once had met Mimi. When we were going to school, we had taken Mimi with us when we went beer drinking at The Pretzel Bell. Mimi had been alone, as Tom was in the army and stationed in Japan, so Ruth had invited Mimi to accompany us. It was only after Ruth reminded me that I vaguely remembered the meeting.

Ruth had not spoken to Mimi in almost a year, but now she was anxious to get hold of her. However, Mimi lived in California and there was a time difference of three hours between us. By 7:00PM our time, Ruth couldn't wait any longer, so she picked up the phone and dialed Mimi's number.

"Hello, Mimi, this is Ruth. I haven't heard from you in such a long time. How are you?" There followed a long conversation bringing each other up to date on family matters and mutual friends.

After the initial, lengthy surge of dialogue between them, Ruth said, "Listen, Mimi, the reason I am calling is to invite you to a wedding." There was a loud reaction on the other end.

"Who's wedding? Mine."

More reaction on the other end. Ruth responded, "Jay Carp."

Again a noisy pause. "Yes, the same one. We went out as a threesome once while Tom was in Japan."

More talk from the other end. "No, his wife died and he was on his way to live in California. He stopped in Ann Arbor to see my mother and it started over again for both of us. I want you to be my bridesmaid."

More phone conversation. "We have to be married in less than two weeks. No shotgun just something connected with his retirement. We will fly to Lake Tahoe whenever you can be there."

"Oh, poop. Hold the phone a second, Mimi." Ruth turned to me and said, "They are leaving tomorrow for a five day stay in The Caribbean and then they are going to Florida to see Tom's family. Damn it, it won't work out."

They talked for a few more minutes and then Ruth hung up. She was disappointed and angry. "Oh shit, what are we going to do now? I just hate the thought of eloping in a shabby ceremony. And I wanted Mimi to be there so badly."

I patted her shoulder and said, "I am not sure of anything yet, Ladybug. Let's see what we can do."

I looked at the list of states again and noticed that Florida did not require a blood test or a waiting period. Maybe all was not lost. "I wonder when Mimi and Tom will be in Florida, and where will they be? Why couldn't we get married in Florida?"

We talked about it for a while and Ruth admitted that it was a possibility. Ruth phoned Mimi again and found the dates they would be in Florida, and where they would be staying. They would be in St. Petersburg in about a week. Ruth wrote the information down, and she told Mimi she would call her back if we could work something out.

St. Petersburg looked like a good possibility. I had friends who had retired in St. Petersburg. I had worked with two of them for over twenty years. During that time we had become personal friends and I could not think of any nicer people to turn to for help. I called one of them, Tom Kehoe, and our opening conversation was almost identical to Ruth's phone call with Mimi. When I explained why we had no later than a two-week deadline, he asked what he could do.

I told him, "Tom, I have never been in the State of Florida. I need information about obtaining a marriage license in St. Petersburg. Ruth and I won't be getting married until near the end of our two-week window because we have a lot to do up here before the wedding and her bridesmaid won't be available for about a week. Once we obtain the marriage license there won't be much time to meet the deadline. Tomorrow, can you call around and get me some information? I will call you back sometime tomorrow afternoon and you can tell me what you found out."

Tom said that he would be delighted to help us but that he needed to know what specific information he was to obtain. I told him to find out where the licenses were purchased, how much they cost, what paperwork would be required for a divorcee and a widower to marry, and if the ceremony could take place immediately after the license was issued. Tom said he would start calling first thing in the morning, and we hung up. He called me back the next day and gave me the details of everything that I had asked him for.

As soon as I finished talking to Tom, Ruth called Mimi back and told her that we would meet them in Florida. She confirmed the time they would arrive in St. Petersburg, their address and their phone number. Mimi asked Ruth if she wanted to know the name of the hotel in the Caribbean where she would be staying just in case Ruth had more information to give her. Ruth laughed and said that she did not need it; she would see them in Florida.

While we were groping for out of state answers, we started grappling with our local problems. We were not sure what personal records we would need. We gathered both of our birth certificates, Virginia's death certificate, Ruth's divorce decree, the GTE retirement papers, and whatever other documents we thought we would need. Within a day or two, Ruth decided that she needed to take some extra time off from work to help get everything done.

She startled me, a day later, by asking me

if I had decided on what type of wedding ring I wanted. I asked, "Do I have a choice?"

"Only as to the type," she replied. "As for whether you are going to wear one or not, there is no question."

I asked, "Why am I being ordered around?"

"Two reasons," she hugged me and then continued, "The first one is the most important one for me. If I am going to take that lousy last name of yours, I want the world to know that you are mine and that I am yours. The second reason is that my first husband was a snake. He never wore his and that hurt me."

I said, "I guess that settles that. I sure hope you pick me out a nice one."

We went into almost every jewelry store in Ann Arbor looking for wedding rings for both of us. I figured that, as soon as Ruth made her choice, I would get a simple, plain band to match. But Ruth had trouble picking out a wedding ring. After looking in most of the good jewelry stores, she still couldn't come to any decision. We were sitting in the parking lot at Briarwood Mall, when I finally got exasperated and asked, "Ruth, what is the problem. You seem to be having a hard time finding anything that suits you."

She turned, and looked at me, I could see

tears forming in her eyes. I felt bad that I had raised my voice. She spoke so quietly and so wistfully that I almost didn't hear her.

"Honey, I don't mean to be such a pain in the ass, but I just can't seem to choose a wedding ring. The last time I did this, I had to pay for both wedding bands and I could not afford an engagement ring, and I always wanted an engagement ring. I know it is silly, but for some reason, I can't get that out of my mind. Let's go back and I will just pick out any wedding ring that you like."

"No, let's go back and pick out a wedding set that you like. You are an aggravation, you are a total pain in the ass, but I absolutely adore you. Why didn't you tell me that you wanted an engagement ring? Let's go do it; let's go get an engagement ring. You are holding up my wedding."

Ruth was hesitant. She said, "Honey, can we afford it?"

"Ladybug, that should not be your concern until I tell you that it is my concern. Yes, we can afford it. My money is to please us, you and me. Only what is left, if there is any left, is my children's inheritance. Come on, turkey, we have to get to Florida."

It did not take Ruth very long to pick out her set of rings, and I selected a plain silver wedding band.

Within the next few days we flew down to Ft. Myers and spent the night with a friend of Ruth's who had lived next door to her in Ypsilanti, for years. The next morning we drove to Sarasota. We got there early in the afternoon, and the first thing we did was to go to the courthouse and apply for a marriage license. While we were standing at the counter filling out the forms, a handsome couple was taking their marriage vows right beside us. The bride wore a beautiful, white wedding gown and the groom was dressed in a gray tuxedo. It was sad because the office noises intruded upon the ceremony, and the nervous couple had to repeat their words several times in order to be heard. Ruth looked at me, and I knew what she was thinking. That was not the way she wanted to marry me.

After we got the license, we picked out a motel. We drove by one that looked very clean, with a fresh coat of paint and a well kept pool. It looked attractive. So, we checked in, unloaded our luggage, and went to dinner. The motel was a disaster. What we did not realize, until we got back from a leisurely meal on Long Boat Key, was that the walls were thinner than our bed sheets. We could hear everything in the rooms on either side of us. We lay in bed and just laughed at our predicament. Ruth whispered in my ear,

"No matter what I told you in the restaurant, we are not doing it tonight." Then she started giggling.

I answered, "If that's the way you are going to be, don't bother to look for any extra money on the bureau. Listen let's check out of here, first thing in the morning."

When we awoke, in the morning, while we cooed and clucked Ruth whispered, "Jay, I don't want to stand at a counter to get married. Don't check out. That is not as important to me as it is to find a nice place for our wedding, even if that means we have to stay dry for a couple of nights. Would you be terribly upset?"

"Not enough to leave you, Ladybug. Come on let's go see about doing this correctly."

On the way out, I stopped by the motel office to tell them that we were almost out of toilet paper and there was no spare roll in our bathroom.

Our search was discouraging. The marriage chapels listed in the yellow pages were dingy marriage mills that ground out weddings commercially, not romantically. Most of them were located in dilapidated sections of the town. The hunt took all day and, as we drove back to the motel late in the afternoon, we were both very quiet and subdued. What made us laugh at first, and then feel even worse, was that we found that the motel had left us half a roll of toilet paper as a spare. We both felt depressed when we left to go eat.

We went back to our restaurant on Long Boat Key which had a marvelous view of the water and good food. Ruth was apprehensive; she waited until we had klunked, and then she asked, "What are we going to do, Jay? I don't want to be married in that busy office unless it is necessary."

Knowing her concern, I tried to answer honestly, "I am not sure yet, Honey. But let's start over. Tomorrow, we will go back to where we got the license and ask the clerks for suggestions."

The next morning we were at the courthouse just as it opened for business. I went inside while Ruth stayed in the car. I was not too optimistic, but we had to start somewhere. I walked up to the counter and approached the youngest looking clerk, hoping that being young would make her more sympathetic towards all lovebirds, no matter what their age.

"Excuse me," I said, "I would like some help, if you can provide it. My lady and I want to get married, but we don't just want to stand at this counter. We looked around yesterday, and all the advertised marriage chapels looked shabby. Do you know of anyplace where we could be married that is attractive?"

"Gosh," she replied, "I don't know of any place around here, but let me ask the other ladies."

She came back in a few minutes with one of the older office clerks. I thought, "So much for my theory of youth and love". The older woman said to me, "I understand your problem. I really don't know why so many couples get married in this office. It is noisy and commercial in here. A niece of mine got married a few weeks ago. I did not attend the ceremony, but I know that it was held at the Selby Gardens. You might try there."

No one in the office could give me directions to the Selby Gardens, so I left and went back to the car.

"Any luck, Honey?" Ruth asked as I got in.

"I am not sure, but I do know that we have a lead. One of the women told me that her niece got married in a place called the Selby Gardens. So, off we go to find it."

I saw a police cruiser parked by the side of the road and the cop told us where the gardens were located and the best way to get there. The Selby Gardens turned out to be a botanical garden facing Sarasota Bay and located close to where we were. When we pulled into the parking lot, we had to sit in the car for a half hour waiting for it to open. After we entered we found a semi-tropical paradise of trees, fish, birds, and flowers. Ruth absolutely came alive at its beauty. She held my hand tightly as we walked around. She asked me two or three times, "Oh, Jay, do you really think we can get married in this garden? Can we afford it? Who do we talk to?"

After we finished our tour, we began to find out about renting the garden. We ended up in the office of the garden manager, discussing terms, price, availability, and what we had to do to rent it for our wedding. Ruth and I reserved the garden, before it opened to the public, from 9:00 to 10:00AM, on Monday, February 1. That was four days away. We finally had the place to have our wedding.

When I paid the manager the one hundred and fifty-dollar rental fee, he told me that, included in the rental, was a free tour of the gardens after the wedding, for anyone associated with the wedding. I thanked him for that information, and told him that I would pass that on to our guests. However, at present, I had more urgent business. I asked him if he could recommend anyone to perform the ceremony. He gave me the name, and the phone number, of a notary public who had done many weddings at the gardens. Ruth and I thanked him, and, on the way to the car, Ruth put her arm around my waist. That surprised me, because Ruth usually was not demonstrative in public.

"Jay, maybe it will work out," she said as she squeezed me.

"Ladybug, it will work out because we are going to make it work out. By the time we leave here, we will be married, and at least one of us will be happy about it."

"God, you are cocky, Jay. What makes you so damn sure of yourself?"

"Damn it Ruth, I am neither cocky nor sure of myself. But look at what has been done during the week or so that you and I have been working on this. We have the rings, the bridesmaid, the license, the location, and the time for the marriage. What we have left to do is to find someone to perform the ceremony, flowers probably, and whatever else you would like or need. And we have the rest of today, all day Friday, all day Saturday and all day Sunday if we need the time, to get ready for the wedding on Monday. Won't you admit that we are in pretty good shape?"

She patted my arm and said, "When you put it that way, I guess you are right. You don't take 'no' for an answer, do you? I am glad that you are in charge and not me. What do we do next?"

"Well," I said, "Let's drive over to St. Armand's Key and see if we can locate a notary public by the name of Ms. Talbert. We will figure out what comes next, after we see her. Please don't forget that we are going out to eat tonight with my friends who got us the information about our wedding license. Maybe we ought to grab a quick snack, but it is getting a little late for us to eat a big lunch."

We drove over to St. Armand's Key and parked. We were amazed; all the main streets of this business area came together at the hub of a circle, and the hub itself is a delightful tourist trap with unique and expensive shops and restaurants.

We found Ms. Talbert's office, on the second floor, over one of the stores around the circle. There was a sign saying that she was out but that she would return after 4:00PM.

"Should we hang around here and wait for her, Jay? There are some really nifty shops we could look at."

I answered, "And that is just the reason we should not hang around. No, Ladybug if we do wait it will make us late for this evening. Besides, we have something else we should do. We have to find a restaurant and make luncheon reservations for a reception after the wedding."

"Are you thinking of Marina Jack's?" Ruth

asked. We had eaten lunch there the previous day and we had enjoyed both the food and the view of the Bay from the restaurant windows. And, equally as important, it was very close to Selby Gardens.

"Yes I was, unless you have any objection," I replied.

"Oh no, Honey, I think that is fine; I liked it very much. But, it seems to me that you are spending quite a bit of money on this wedding. Our rings, plane tickets, car rental, motel, restaurants, and the wedding itself. Can we really afford it?"

"Listen Ruth, I know that you have had to scrimp for years. But, if I am not concerned about spending buckies, you should not be either. I want this to be a happy wedding for each of us. Whatever it costs to get this wedding accomplished is what it will cost. So, quit worrying."

For once, Ruth did not try to have the last word. She just kissed me.

We stopped by Marina Jack's and reserved a table for twelve to fifteen for lunch on Monday, February 1st. I asked them to try and make sure that it was one of the tables that overlooked the water.

We went back to our thin walled motel, checked to make sure that they had not given our reserve half roll of toilet paper to someone else, and then I made two phone calls. The first was to my brokerage firm in Boston, and I arranged for them to send me a new supply of money and to have it here by Friday.

The second call was to Ms. Talbert. She answered the phone and, after a brief conversation, she told me that she was available on February 1st. I spelled out my full name and made an appointment to see her, tomorrow morning at 9:00AM.

Ruth heard both of these conversations and, although she did not like me withdrawing so much money, she was pleased that our plans were beginning to take shape.

That evening, we went out to eat with Mary Anne and Bill Stevens, and Maureen and Tom Kehoe. Not only had Bill, Tom, and I worked together, but Mary Anne had also worked for GTE. She had been a secretary in our group. The four of them had known Virginia and me for many years and her death had shocked and saddened them.

Ruth didn't tell me but I sensed that she was apprehensive about meeting my friends. She was concerned because they had been friends of Virginia and she was nervous about what they would think of her. After giving it some thought, I decided not to say anything. I had no doubt that they would like her, they are very friendly, warmhearted people. But telling her that would not ease her anxieties. She would have see for herself.

After the initial introductions were made, and the awkwardness of meeting someone new was over, we all had a drink or two and relaxed. It was a hot evening and I took off my jacket and left it on the back of a chair. Unfortunately, I forgot to retrieve the jacket when we went out to eat at a steakhouse.

While we were eating at the restaurant, the significance of not having my jacket dawned on me; my wallet was still in the inside pocket. I told Tom and Bill that they would have to lend me some money so that Ruth and I could continue to eat. They ribbed me unmercifully, as well they should, and they were enjoying themselves at my expense. After all, the four of them had put up with me for twenty years. Everyone, except Ruth and I, thought that my mistake was funny. I was embarrassed and Ruth was more than a little angry with me.

When we returned to Tom's house, I paid him back, and took a lot more ribbing. The four of them completely surprised Ruth and me by bringing out a bottle of champagne and a cake in our honor. They poured each of us a glass and insisted that I make a toast. I walked over to Ruth, put my arm around her waist, touched champagne glasses with her and said, "Klunk, I love you Ruth."

Then, I turned and said, "Here is to old friends and new love." I cried a little.

We spent hours talking; they all insisted on telling her about some of my escapades when we had been working together. Before we left, Maureen and Mary Anne told Ruth where to get flowers for the wedding. They also insisted that they wanted to bring the wedding cake.

When we went out the door, we all kissed and hugged one another. Ruth was very quiet on the drive back to the motel. When we pulled into the parking lot, she said, "Two things impressed me tonight. The first is that they are such nice people. They made me feel at home. I really had a good time.

"The second thing is that I have never heard such stories about work in all of my life. If those stories are true, and I guess they are, how you kept your job without getting fired is a mystery to me. Your bosses seemed to put up with a lot from you."

I laughed as I said, "Ruth, all those stories that they told you are true and there are others that they don't even know about. You have to remember that I worked for GTE for over thirty years. In all those years, whether I was a half ass engineer or a half ass manager, I followed three rules. The first was to work hard; the second was to tell the truth; and the third was to have a good time. And I told everyone who worked for me that I expected him, or her, to follow those same rules.

"There were times when I was in conflict with everyone, my bosses, the Air Force, even my co-workers. That was not important. What was important to me was that, at the end of the day, I could honestly say that I had done the best I could.

"What saved me from management's wrath was that I knew what had to be done and I knew how to get it done. Those abilities made them put up with my approach to work. Depending upon your point of view, I was either a devil or a delight."

Ruth just shook her head and smiled as she said, "Someday, you will have to write a book about your work. Maybe then I will be able to understand the whole bunch of you."

***

Friday morning we drove over to St. Armand's circle early, and sat outdoors at a café, eating Danish pastries and sipping coffee. The air was bright and warm from the sunshine, and that seemed to make the aromas that arose from the flowers, the coffee, and the baked goods, all the more enticing. We sat, holding hands, at peace as individuals, and content as a couple.

We walked up the stairs to Ms. Talbert's office just before nine, and introduced ourselves to the small, vivacious woman sitting at her desk. We talked generalities for awhile, got on a first name basis, and then began discussing our wedding. We told her of our arrangements, and asked if she would perform the service. I left to get coffee for all of us and, when I returned, Ruth was amused and was laughing.

After I sat down, she shook her head at me and said, "Now I know what you have been through all of your life, and what awaits me. Nancy did not think anyone would show up this morning. She had written your name down as Jay Crap." Ruth slowly and carefully spelled it out,"C-R-A-P. She thought that someone was playing a stupid prank on her."

I sighed and said, "Nancy, that name has always caused me grief. I try to be careful when I pronounce it and spell it. I am sorry if you misunderstood me."

Nancy was a little embarrassed, but it really was no problem for me as I had been facing this dilemma all of my life. Ruth had originally protested a little about getting a last name like

Carp when she agreed to marry me. But when I had offered to take her maiden name of Ormondroyd as our last name instead she declined, saying that, if she were going to marry me, she was going to take my last name.

When we were through with our discussions, I asked Nancy if she knew of anyone who could sing at our wedding. She made two phone calls, and gave us a sheet of paper with a name and address written on it. She said, "He's available, and he has a marvelous voice. He will be home until noon, if you are interested."

We drove over to his house and he sang a couple of songs for us. He really did possess a magnificent voice. We engaged him on the spot and the three of us selected the two songs he would sing.

Then, we went to find the local Smith Barney office because my money was held in a fund growing in their financial garden. We got a fresh supply of money and drove back to our motel. I made a phone call to find out which gate Ruth and I would use to get into the Selby Gardens at 8:45 Monday morning and then Ruth made a phone call to the florist to insure that she would get the proper corsage delivered on time Monday. That completed all of our wedding arrangements, we had nothing else to do for the wedding except to show up at the Selby Gardens. We could now stop worrying about a spare roll of toilet paper and check out; that was a pleasure for both of us.

After we had put the luggage in the car, Ruth came over to me and said, "Honey, everything is arranged and taken care of. I didn't think it was possible, but it's done. I am so happy." Words I enjoyed hearing.

\*\*\*

We drove across Florida to the East Coast and spent Friday night with some friends of mine who had moved to Ormond Beach. I have known Vincent and Marilyn Petrie for thirty years and, throughout all of this time, they have been cheerfully disagreeing with, and cheerfully correcting, each other. Interruptions didn't bother them, they just continue talking and have happily accepted one another without getting upset. They are great fun to be with and Ruth felt comfortable with them. We both pleaded with them to come to our wedding, but they had other plans and could not attend. All four of us were disappointed.

Saturday, we went to Melbourne Beach, and visited Ruth's cousin, Arlene Hoopes, and her husband, Bob. Ruth and Arlene are about the same age and they hadn't seen each other since they were thirteen years old. The last time was when Ruth went back to Philadelphia with her mother to visit her mother's parents and relatives. There was a lot of simultaneous talking between Ruth and Arlene as they attempted to catch up on their family history during those intervening years. After breakfast, just before we left, we also invited them to our wedding but they also had previous commitments and wouldn't be able to attend. We didn't do too well in recruiting attendees for our wedding.

We returned to Sarasota on Sunday afternoon and checked into a big hotel on the Ringling Causeway. Ruth came into the hotel with me, and after I had registered, she asked, "Did you lock the car when we came in?"

I was a little surprised as I thought that she was checking on me. "Yes, I most certainly did."

She then asked, "Is it blocking someone's way?"

I was a little annoyed because I still thought that she was checking on me. "No, PITA, it is not blocking anyone's way."

"Good. Let's go up and make sure the room is not like the last one we stayed in." I was no longer annoyed. We got on the elevator and pushed the button for our room on the top floor. When we were alone on the elevator, she said,

"All this talk about getting married is making me horny."

We really didn't spend much time checking the room. The result of our hasty entry was that I did not compare the clock in the room against my wristwatch. Usually, the very first thing I did whenever I entered a new room was to check the hotel room clock. I developed this habit because I traveled so much when I was working and I needed to be on time for the dispatches to the missile sites.

Early in the evening, Ruth called Mimi to make sure that she and Tom were at his family's home. They chatted a good long time, and Ruth asked them to be at our door by 7:30 AM. She gave Mimi the name of our hotel and the room number.

Sunday evening, before we went to sleep, I set the alarm so that we would be awake in plenty of time to get ready in the morning. Of course, we both had a fitful night, cuddling, talking, dozing, waking, and trying to get back to sleep.

After the alarm went off, we showered together, and began to dress. We prepared and preened and finally, we were ready. Mimi and Tom had assured us that they would be at the door to our room by 7:30 A.M. We sat and nervously waited for them to arrive. When the clock in the room read quarter to eight, Ruth began to get restive.

"This is not like Mimi and Tom to be late. Especially on a day like today," she said.

For the first time, I looked at my wristwatch and then at the alarm clock. "Oh shit, Honey," I said loudly, "it is only 6:00AM." I called the desk to confirm the time. Our room clock was set incorrectly.

Ruth said, "Poop."

"Ladybug, I am sorry. I should have checked the clock. We have plenty of time to wait until they arrive, what do you want to do?"

She laughed, with that deep pleasant laugh of hers, waved her finger at me, and said, "Forget what you are thinking Jay, I do not want to get mussed up. Here is what we are going to do." She brought out our book of Sunday New York Times crossword puzzles. We were sitting on the sofa, working on one of them, when Mimi and Tom arrived at the time they were supposed to, just before 7:30 AM.

We went for coffee and Ruth and Mimi seemed to talk at the same time until it was time to go to the Selby Gardens. The wedding went off smoothly. It was a small party of about eleven or twelve friends; the view of the bay was magnificent; the weather was clear and cool; and Ruth and I and several others were teary eyed.

194

After the wedding, we invited everyone to tour the grounds of this lovely garden, explaining that they would be allowed to look around even though it would not be open to the public for another half-hour. We told them that we would meet them at Marina Jack's at noontime.

In the meantime, Ruth and I had some errands that we needed to run. We took the signed, notarized copy of the marriage certificate to the courthouse, and got the marriage license certified. Then, we got copies of each certified document and addressed them to the appropriate people, specifically by name, within GTE. We went to the post office and sent the documents and the signed papers asking for early retirement, in a large envelope, marked special delivery, registered, return receipt requested. We had beaten our deadline. After that, we rejoined our guests at Marina Jack's and celebrated our wedding day.

\*\*\*

We left Florida, and flew back to Michigan on the following Wednesday. For the first week after we got home Ruth and I were inundated with phone calls, visitors, and mail, congratulating us and wishing us well. Ruth's daughters came over frequently to hear all the details of the trip and especially the details of the wedding. One of our friends had video taped the wedding and they watched it again and again. They were happy for me, and absolutely delighted for their mother.

After the initial inrush of interest, Ruth went back to work and our routine continued in exactly the same pattern as it had been before our wedding. We were comfortable with each other.

Our closeness had some startling effects. Occasionally, we appeared to be in two time zones at the same time; we would ping pong between the past and the present. Ideas, thoughts, and memories merged, mingled, and meshed, like a kaleidoscope, and yesterday would suddenly appear with today. It was an odd phenomenon.

Out of a clear blue-sky one day, Ruth asked me, "Did you know that when we first dated you never wore anything but white socks?"

"Yes, I remember," I told her. I had always worn white socks. That was all I ever had known while I was growing up. It was after we broke up, and I started working, that I began to match the colors of my socks with my business clothes.

I was watching Ruth as she was making

out a grocery list one morning. She was writing with a blue ball point pen.

"Did you know that you never used any pen other than a green ink pen when we dated?" She stopped writing and looked at me. "No," she said, "I don't remember that at all."

"It's true, Ladybug," I replied.

About two weeks later, Ruth was looking in her recipe box for a dish that she wanted to make. She called me over and said, "Honey, you were right. Look at the color of the ink on these old recipes. It's funny that you should remember that."

All of her old recipe cards were written with green ink.

Lying in bed naked, one morning, I recalled something that she had said to me so many years ago and I turned and started looking at her breasts.

Ruth asked, after a few minutes, "Jay, why are you staring at my boobs?"

I answered, "I remember that you and I went to Whitmore Lake on a hot, Sunday afternoon, while we were going to school. You wore a two piece bathing suit and I said something about you having a beautiful figure. You told me then, that your right one was bigger than your left one. I looked, and looked but, with your bathing suit on, I couldn't tell if one was really bigger than the other. I decided that you were probably correct but that no one else could possibly notice any difference. Even now, looking at you naked, I can't see any difference."

"Jay, I can't believe I would ever say anything to you about my boobs. Are you sure that this conversation occurred?"

"Well, Ruth, don't you believe that your left one is smaller than your right?"

"Yes, I have always been embarrassed about that, but I just can't believe that I would ever tell you, or any one else about something so personal."

Ruth was not the slightest bit prudish, but back in the Forties and Fifties, personal privacy included body functions and sex. Menstrual cycles were not forecast and broadcast like weather reports, and communal confessions about sex positions and masturbation were not loudly and proudly trumpeted in public. Even now, Ruth did not care what words I used to name either our body parts or our sex acts, but she herself would only use certain terms. Her breasts were never titties or tits; they were boobies or boobs. Likewise, she did not use either of the words pussie or cunt for her vagina; that was her "Hmm Hmm." She never told me where she got that name.

Similarly, she would not discuss our sex

activities with anyone. Both Robin and Christie would have been delighted to hear about what we were doing while Tracy did not even want to think about her mother having sex. Whatever their attitudes, Ruth was too private a person to consider saying anything to them, or any one else.

Sometimes, while I was sleeping, I would dream about our past and I would wake up completely disoriented. For a second, I would be dazed, and not know where I was. Then I would hear the sound of Ruth breathing and I would recall the present. I would lie there and be thankful that we were both alive and had known each other twice. I would lean over, kiss whatever part of Ruth was closest to me, and go back to sleep. I don't know why, but I never told Ruth about these early morning kisses.

\*\*\*

After we had been married two months, I began to have some second thoughts about our marriage ceremony. We had gone out to eat by ourselves one evening and Ruth asked me why I was so quiet.

"Because I have been thinking," I said.

"Should I be worried?" she asked.

"Yes, Wife, I think you should," I answered

her. "I have been thinking and I have decided that we should be in 'The Guiness Book of Records'. You will probably have to quit your job so you can help."

She looked skeptical as she asked, "And just how are you getting us into the record book?"

"Easy as pie," I replied. "You quit your job, we get married in each of the forty nine other states, and, presto, we have set a record."

"And you are completely off your rocker," she said as she started to grin.

"Well, that may be," I concede, "But two things will happen. We will go down in history as the most married couple in the world and you won't be able to afford 50 divorce lawyers."

Ruth was laughing, and shaking her head, "Honey, you have absolutely nothing to worry about. First of all, I am not about to kill the fatted calf. And secondly, divorce is out of the question. As is being married in fifty states."

Since I was half joking, I did not pursue my idea any further and we did not set any record. Now that she is gone, I wish we had.

One morning, Ruth started our coo and cluck session by saying, "Honey, it is time that we go see a lawyer."

I replied, "Absolutely not, no way."

She was surprised, "Jay, why not?"

"Because it is much too soon for a divorce."

Ruth laughed, "Silly. I am not thinking of a divorce, at least not quite yet. What I am thinking is that we ought to take the correct steps to make sure that your money goes to your girls and my money, such as it is, goes to my girls."

We had had talks about our finances many times, but we never did anything after our discussions. It was not that we disagreed, it was more a case of mutual disinterest. Neither of us wanted the other's purse.

I had asked Ruth, at one time before we were married, if she wanted a prenuptial agreement. She told me that I probably needed one more than she did, because I had a lot more money. She said that if I trusted her, than she certainly trusted me. That was all right with me because Ruth was honest to a fault; up until that point, our basis for doing business with each other was our trust.

She was right, though, about us setting up trusts and living wills. We needed to make our financial parade march to the right beat so that we could pass in revue without having the government grab our money. As it turned out, when we did consult a lawyer, her approach to dividing her assets was slightly different than mine. Some of the difference was due to our relationship as husband and wife, and some of it was due to her experience with her father's estate.

Because her father had not liked Ruth's husband, he left all of his money in a trust, to be inherited by Ruth's daughters when Ruth died. She got a small yearly sum, but the bulk of his estate was made totally unavailable to her. During the years of raising her girls in hard financial times, that money would have made Ruth's life easier. She was not bitter about it, but she vowed that any money she had would go directly to her children.

Her mother's estate, which would prove to be larger than her father's, was to go to Ruth. But, by the time she finally did inherited her mother's estate, she didn't have any financial concerns. We were married and we had enough money to live well. However, what she had been through taught her what she was going to do with her estate. What Ruth wanted was simple; all of her assets were to be divided in three equal amounts to go to her daughters.

On the other hand, I had no family inheritances to be concerned about. Whatever I had, had been gathered during my lifetime. I wanted my money divided equally among my girls, but I also had another concern. I wanted to make sure that Ruth lived comfortably for the rest of her life if I passed away first. She would have very little of her own money until her mother died, and, if her mother outlived me, Ruth would be in dire straights. I felt that insuring her well being was absolutely my first priority.

Whatever I had left, after I was through using it, would go to my kids. I never considered that my assets were to be spent grudgingly so that my children could have more. However, a portion of my estate would be available for Ruth until she passed away. Then the remainder would revert over to my girls. I wanted full use for Ruth and me, and then, when she and I could no longer spend money, they would have their chance to do it for me.

***

It was not until after we were married that I finally got to meet two of Ruth's closest friends, Dick and Dottie Bauer. Dottie and Ruth had known each other for years. And, in a way, meeting them opened the final doors to the closets of secrecy between Ruth and me.

Ruth and Dottie first met when they were on the same bowling team and for years, the two of them had gone to bowling tournaments, cruised bars, and raised hell together. When Dottie met and married Dick, the equation became different, but they still kept in close contact.

Why it took so long before I met them, I do not know. Ruth introduced me to her other friends and acquaintances almost as fast as she could dial the telephone. At one point, after I first returned, I began to think that I was on display. She would mention Dick and Dottie and say that I had to meet them, and then go on to another subject. Of course, they were extremely busy in their own right. Dick was an executive with Ford Motor Company, and Dottie worked in a doctor's office, and they had their own active social and family life. Whatever the reasons, it took a while before the four of us got together.

I liked them immediately. Dick and Dottie are both warm hearted and honest. As individuals they put you at ease and as a couple they charm you with their grace and hospitality. The four of us hit it off, and we were comfortable with one another.

The first time we met we went out to dinner on a Saturday night, and, after our meal, we came back to Dick and Dottie's house for after dinner drinks. With Dick and Dottie, that meant drinking Dottie's extra strong black Russians until three or four in the morning. Dottie wanted to hear all the details of how we first had met, and, the more we drank, the more questions she asked.

Since these were Ruth's friends, I let her do the talking while I quietly drank and listened. She enjoyed telling Dottie about the bus stop, my fraternity brothers, and my not speaking to her. As she continued to talk, though, I began to pay more attention because she added some details to the story that I had never heard before.

Ruth said, "After a while, I was determined to meet him and make him talk to me. It made me mad that all of his fraternity brothers would engage me in conversation but that he wouldn't bother to speak to me."

She stopped speaking and looked directly at me. When we were locked in eye contact, she smiled, and continued, "I was furious with you for not talking to me, and not noticing me in that class that we were both taking. On the day we met, I rushed out of the nearest exit door, ran down the steps to the door you used, and I made sure that you bumped into me."

All four of us laughed. Dottie, of course, wanted to know why I had been such a slow leak. I couldn't give her any real reason, so we had another round of black Russians to toast Ruth's actions. We all had such a good time that it continued until almost daybreak Sunday morning. Ruth and I both woke up, around noon, with hangovers, and it wasn't until almost 6:00PM that I began to feel better. It had been quite an evening.

Two or three days later, during one of our coo and cluck sessions, I said, "Wife, you absolutely took me by surprise at Dick and Dottie's. I did not know that you had bumped into me on purpose and you never told me that you were angry that I never spoke to you. In fact, I never knew that you had such a quick temper until I returned to see your mother."

She replied, "Honey, back then I just never displayed my temper. Besides, I don't have to tell you everything, do I?"

"No, I guess not. There should be room for privacy. But why tell Dick and Dottie when you won't tell me?"

Ruth giggled, and then answered, "I don't even know why I told that to Dottie, except that I knew she would understand. I think I had forgotten about it until those black Russians stirred my memory.

"But I really was mad. I thought that you were a big, handsome hunk and you wouldn't even say 'Hello'. That had never happened to me before, so, I decide to do something about it. What I can't figure out is why you were so shy until I made the first move. Can you tell me why?"

I nuzzled her neck, and kissed her on the cheek. "Ruth, I didn't grow up until years after we broke up. I finally discovered that I was hiding from myself. After that, I realized that I had to stand up and be honest. It sounds simple, but it took me years to figure it out.

"I didn't try to tell you about myself when we first met, because I just didn't know how. I was afraid of losing you, and as a result of my fear, I did lose you.

"I wouldn't have used that word, 'shy', although you might be correct. I would have said that I was afraid of not being liked or accepted. I was frightened of what people would think of me.

"Let me tell you a story that I have never told anyone before because I have been so embarrassed by it for years." And that was when I told Ruth about my house catching fire every Saturday afternoon. After I finished telling her about our bed bugs, I realized that the memories were now more humorous than hurtful, and I began to tell her about other events that had bothered me.

For the first time, I told her about my mother who loved to play beano, our shabby homes, and my problems when I was going to school. Ruth had a hard time believing that my mother could leave her children alone in the car for four or five hours at a time. She held me tightly and told me how sorry she was that she had not understood me better when we were going to school. My wounds had stopped bleeding a long time ago, but my memories needed to be massaged, relaxed and put to rest. And that is what talking with Ruth did for me, it didn't change my upbringing but it did put it into perspective.

By the same token, Ruth also began to tell me what had bothered her as she grew up. Even though I had seen the tension between her mother and father, I had always assumed her family life was better than mine. After all, her father was listed in "Who's Who" and her mother came from an established Philadelphia family.

When Ruth told me the details about her childhood, I was surprised to learn that she had her own deep, dark secrets. Ruth carried about as many childhood scars as I did. For some reason, knowing that we each had painful memories brought us even closer together. I hugged her and ached for her exactly as she ached for me. Loneliness and longing are sad sugars that flavor and sweeten the fruits of love.

When she was young, her mother's attitude troubled Ruth constantly. Mrs. O had always been cold and hard to both Ruth and her brother but she was especially hard on Ruth. She was not pleased that her youngest child had been a girl and not a boy. Ruth grew up feeling guilty and unsure of herself and not understanding why she felt that way.

Once, when Ruth was a young girl, she came home from school late and found that her mother had locked her out of the house as a punishment for walking slowly and being late. Ruth knocked on the door and pleaded to be let in but her mother kept the door locked. Soon, Ruth had to go the bathroom and she begged her mother to unlock the door and let her use the toilet. All to no avail, her mother would not relent. Ruth wet her pants and had to stay outside in her soiled clothes until her mother decided it was time to unlock the door. Her mother finally allowed her in, scolded her for being late, and spanked her for wetting her pants.

From the age of ten, until she was thirteen years old, Ruth was chubby. When her mother was entertaining guests, she would call Ruth into the room, and then she would introduce Ruth as my fat daughter. This would embarrass Ruth terribly, and she asked her mother not to speak like that in front of company. It did her no good and her mother continued to demean Ruth publicly and privately.

Her father had gone into the Navy during World War II. Years later, he asked Ruth if she thought that he had abandoned her. She had never given that any thought, as she was young then, and all the men were going into the armed forces. Her father told her that he had gone into the navy primarily to get away from his wife.

When he told her about wanting to escape from his wife, it did not come as any surprise to Ruth, and it did not upset her. She understood that the constant baiting and insults that he had been subjected to would have been enough to drive him out of the house. It was in the twilight of his life when he told Ruth that, on his wedding night, he learned that he had made a mistake. Poor Jessie Ormondroyd, neither Ruth nor I could figure out why he never got a divorce.

As Ruth matured into a young woman there began an uneasy peace between her mother and her because Ruth was not the primary target of her mother's cold wrath. Ruth's father was. Occasionally, her mother still lashed out at Ruth, but for the most part, there was a cool, civil truce between them while her mother sniped at her father. During the time I was going with Ruth, she never mentioned her hostility towards her mother, but the strained relationships among the three of them were obvious. Back then, she and I did our best to avoid discussions about our respective families.

When she was younger, Ruth was jealous that her brother Edward had gotten out of the house as quickly as he could by joining the navy.

He never came back to the family and was on the West Coast when Ruth and I were going to school. He wrote some charming and successful children's books and settled in upper New York in Trumansburg. He and I met for the first time after Ruth and I got back together.

When Ruth married Mike, her parents expressed their disapproval by refusing to attend the wedding. She had to take care of all the wedding arrangements herself, and it was hard for her to get over the fact that her parents were of no help to her when she needed them.

After her husband started Dental School, at The University of Michigan, Ruth bought her house in Ypsilanti. Ruth told me, that, in many ways, this was the worst period in their relationship. Her mother and father wanted to see Ruth and their grandchildren, but they wanted to have nothing to do with Mike. And, as he started drinking more and whoring more and avoiding his responsibilities, Ruth realized her parents had been right. But what was she to do? She couldn't defend the error that she had made and now she had three young girls to raise and protect. Her parents were very critical, and finally, she had to tell them not to discuss Mike in front of her daughters. For the most part, they complied with her wishes.

Her mother and father were much better

grandparents than they were parents, especially her mother. Her father always was a softhearted person and he liked children, but the change in her mother astonished Ruth. Her mother held the girls, played with them, and even playfully bit them on their butts; something she had not done with either of her children. As a result, Robin, Christie, and Tracy grew up loving their grandparents and never learning of their mother's strange upbringing until they themselves were adults.

When Ruth's mother found out that her husband had made his will so that his money would go to his grandchildren and not Ruth, she called him a jackass and a goddamn fool. Of course, this made him all the more stubborn, and, when he died, in 1974, the money went into escrow until Ruth's death. Her father did not change his will, even though Ruth had gotten divorced in 1968.

After hearing these stories, I understood Ruth's attitudes towards her parents and I became more patient when she said that she hated her mother. As I held her tightly, I told her I would have felt the same way.

***

Ruth called our trip to Florida, "Our wedding

interruption." We returned to the same ebb and flow of our lives as husband and wife, and our new relationship made no difference in our routines. However, since our marriage marked a more formal arrangement than just living together, it did have a subtle effect on some of our long-term plans.

There were two topics about which we had been having on going discussions without ever coming to any conclusions. One had been the house we lived in. I wanted to remodel it—Ruth did not want to remodel. The other was Ruth's job. I wanted Ruth to retire—Ruth did not want to retire.

Ruth had lived in her house for more than thirty-five years. Most of that time, she had been the only adult, and she had her own established patterns and routines. As a result, from her point of view, the house was cozy and livable.

From my point of view, it was neither. It was cramped, cluttered and dark. I considered it a mess. First, the bedroom was just too damn small. I could not get out of the bed on my side, as the bed was against both walls. Once we were in bed, I would either have to crawl over Ruth or shinny down through the foot of the bed and over a hope chest to get out. And with all the furniture in the room, there was no other place for the bed except the corner. I was always apologizing for waking her up, in the middle of the night, just to go to the bathroom. Ruth did not seem to care about being awakened, but it annoyed me. Why should I have to make an announcement every time I needed to go to the bathroom?

The bathroom itself was another minor irritant between us. It was small and Ruth had it jammed with creams, unguents, cosmetics and other feminine paraphernalia leaving no room for my razor, shaving cream, after-shave lotion, and other masculine paraphernalia. We found ourselves pawing through each other's things, muttering about how messy our partner was, while we kept looking for our own stuff. Add to that the fact that Ruth took a long time getting ready, and you have a situation where we would each have to check with the other before using the bathroom for any purpose.

Over the years of being alone, Ruth had developed a habit of either strewing her clothes around or hanging them on the moldings of the bedroom and bathroom doorways. There were three tiny bedrooms and one bathroom, and their doorways faced each other in a very small hall off the dining room. I didn't even have to touch the hangars, as just walking by would cause the hangars and clothes to fall. Even Ruth, who would always caution me before I went near the hangars, had the same problem. After either of us knocked something down, we would swear. I swore the most because knocking clothing down, picking it up, and then replacing it on the door-frame was not my idea of fun and games. It was annoying to Ruth and damn aggravating to me.

Finally, the cellar was a mess. There was a path from the bottom of the cellar stairs over to the washer and dryer located against a wall. The only other pathway was from the stairs to the furnace and the water heater. The rest of the cellar was completely filled with discarded, unused, or broken furniture, appliances that no longer worked, and junk that had been accumulated, and stored, over the years. Nothing that had ever been taken down into the cellar had ever been brought up the stairs again. There was not a square foot of open space. There might have been some usable articles in the cellar, but everything was so stacked and jumbled that it was impossible to move off the two paths.

After I returned from California and saw the cellar, I told Ruth that the basement needed to be cleaned out. Although almost all of my furniture would go to my three daughters after the house was sold, there would be a few pieces that would be shipped to me. The only place we would be able to put them, when they arrived, was in the cellar.

Ruth agreed. She knew the cellar was a

mess but she had been inadvertently trapped. She had paid no attention until it was too late, and then she could not make up her mind how to start a cleanup. She not only was grateful, she also thanked me for making the offer to clean out the mess. Neither of us realized, until after I began, just how dirty a job it was going to be.

After talking with Ruth, I started by getting Richard, Christie's husband, and his truck, over to our house. We hauled some old refrigerators and freezers to the recycling center; no one could recall if they even worked or how long they had been in the cellar. That gave me some working space and then I spent days sorting out furniture and putting things into piles for Ruth to decide what she wanted to do with them. After she determined what she wanted to keep, or what she wanted to give to her daughters, I would donate the rest to charity or throw out what nobody could use. It was dusty and dirty work.

I was halfway finished with the cellar, the massive piles of furniture were beginning to disappear and the floor was beginning to appear, when I found the mother lode of cat shit. For years Ruth's cats, and she had had two or three cats at any given time, had been going down to the back of the cellar and using it as their sandbox. After thirty-five years of making deposits, the entire back third of the cellar floor was covered in about three inches of hardened cat shit. Ruth was absolutely mortified when I showed her that mess; she had had no idea that it was there. I almost had to chisel it to pry it off the floor. Every day when she came home from work, she would come down the cellar to see how I was doing, and she would profusely apologize. Cleaning that mess up was a nasty, slow going chore, and I was glad when I finally finished.

After I had cleaned out the cellar, I would go through the house looking to see if anything could be done to make our lives easier. I thought that the house should be remodeled, and I knew that Ruth did not want to do it. I was sure that making changes would give us more room and make living together easier.

I talked to Ruth about making the house more comfortable. I suggested combining two of the small bedrooms into one large bedroom for our use and adding on a new room in the back of the house. I also wanted to finish off the basement by installing a new bathroom and putting in two large rooms downstairs.

Although Ruth could see the need for change, she was reluctant to do anything. We discussed it for months, and finally, after grudgingly agreeing with me, and consulting with her daughters and her friends, she conceded. The house could be remodeled.

During the five months it took to make these changes, the other topic we had been discussing, her retirement, was completely put aside. All the normal inconveniences associated with re-modeling, the dirt, the noise, the confusion, the delays, were visited upon us. Ruth would go to work early and stay late just so that she would not be involved with this long-term temporary mess. She still had to put up with the construc-tion consequences when she got home; she was not happy and she let me know about it in no uncertain terms. During this transition period, she called the project, "Jay's job."

However, when it was finally finished, and the new room added a lightness to the entire house, and we weren't jousting for the one bath-room, and we could each get out of bed without disturbing the other, Ruth apologized for her attitude. She said she loved our new home. She was delighted to go shopping for new window dressings, new furniture, and new carpeting for the whole house. She would always ask if we could afford what she was buying, and the look of happiness she gave me when I told her to just buy it and stop worrying, delighted me. She had had so little for so long that her happiness was my catnip.

Our discussions about her job were much

more complicated than our discussions about her house. She knew that now, she could quit working any time she wanted, and not have to worry about finances. But she wanted to keep working, at least for a while. She was the office manager at a mental health clinic and she enjoyed her job. She had never been happier than she was now but, in the past, her life had taken surprising twists and turns. Ruth did not like changes. She wanted to work until she got used to her new life.

I could understand that, so I never insisted that she quit her job. I suggested Ruth continue working until she felt that it was time to quit. Sooner or later, Ruth would feel comfortable enough with herself, and her new life to give up working and do only what she wanted to do. It hadn't taken me long to start to enjoy my retirement, and I knew that she would feel the same way once she stopped working. She just needed more time.

***

The fact that Ruth worked limited us from taking long trips. Instead, we went away for weekends. Occasionally, she would take a day of vacation and we would take three-day trips to do whatever we wanted. We saw the fall foliage on the Leelanaw Peninsula, "The Phantom of the

Opera" in Toronto, and we had a jazz weekend in Chicago. We both enjoyed these adventures but Ruth always felt constrained to get back in time to get to work.

One cold, miserable, Sunday, in the middle of winter, we were sitting side by side, working on the Sunday New York Times crossword puzzle. It was dark outside and gloomy inside; we were stuck on a word and both of us were fidgety. All of a sudden, for no reason at all, I asked, "Ladybug, why don't we plan on taking a trip to Alaska this summer?"

A visit to Alaska had always been one of Ruth's dreams. I had not been nearly as enthusiastic about it as Ruth. I had seen my share of ice and snow and cold weather and I wasn't in a rush to see any more. I had spent almost eleven months in Thule, Greenland, and over a year in Grand Forks, North Dakota. Those are cold climates, and I thought that Alaska was just more of the same. So, while I wasn't really opposed to going to Alaska, I was a little indifferent.

"Oh Honey," Ruth replied, "Can we? Can we afford it?"

"I would imagine that if we pack sandwiches to take with us, we should be able to afford it."

She wagged her finger at me and replied, "Don't be such a smartass. I always worry about money. You know that I can't help it."

I said, "I am sorry. I know you are concerned, and that I shouldn't tease you. Your answer is yes, we can afford it. If you are interested, we can go to Alaska this summer."

From that moment on, Ruth enjoyed examining all the travel brochures in detail, talking about the various options, and wallowing in not being able to make up her mind. We finally found a package that we liked and we began to plan our trip.

Our biggest worry was Ruth's mother. She was 85 years old, disoriented, and difficult to communicate with. We had to raise our voices, literally to a scream, to make her understand that we were going on a trip. Every time we told her we were taking a trip she would ask where we were going, and we would answer, "Alaska." She would reply, "Oh, yes, I know where that is and I know the song that they sing about it, 'with a banjo on my knee.'"

Ruth made arrangements with her three daughters to visit their grandmother while we were gone. We were both concerned about her mother. She could pass away while we were travelling, or she could linger for years. We decided not to delay our trip, so, in July of 1994, we went to Alaska.

Two things about that trip made a lasting

impression on us. The first was the primal beauty of that wild country. Alaska is God's anteroom. From the first, as we started up the Inland Passage, the terrain stirred and awed us. All we could say over and over was, "breathtaking." Each natural wonder was constantly replaced by another natural wonder that was even more spectacular. Right from the start, I admitted to Ruth that my concept of Alaska was wrong, and that she was right. She laughed, patted my hand, and refrained from saying, "I told you so."

Our side trips were the frosting on our cake. We took a flight in a pontoon plane to a lake that was absolutely pristine. When we landed, and we were bobbing around in the middle of this lake, we could easily believe that we were the only people in the world. The silence made us speak in hushed tones. We took a train ride up the mountains that the miners had climbed when the Klondike gold rush took place. You could almost feel the fever that gripped and drove them relentlessly, even as you saw what they had to endure in their search for wealth.

We rejoiced in the beauty, but we also wondered how soon before civilization would begin its encroachment and make alterations to this wilderness?

What also surprised me was that we made no friends on this trip. Ordinarily, Ruth could get a tombstone to sing, but not on this trip. Part of the reason we didn't meet anyone we wanted to get to know was because our dining arrangements were a disaster.

The first night at our table of eight, which consisted of four couples, we had problems that continued throughout the entire voyage. One of the couples was an Iranian husband and wife. The man spoke no English and his wife spoke very little and they had a difficult time commnicating with anyone. What compounded their confusion into a serious concern was that they were both orthodox Jews and they had made arrangements to follow their dietary laws. Their children had purchased this tour as a present for their parents, and they had ordered, and paid for a bottle of Champagne for their parent's first meal, and kosher food for the entire trip. The couple received neither, and the woman could not make herself understood when she asked about these prior arrangements. To make matters almost intolerable, they were both treated shabbily by a very haughty steward. Throughout the trip, this couple had problems getting the food that had been promised them, and the waiter and the steward showed absolutely no signs of sympathy or compassion. At one of our final meals, their bottle of Champagne was summarily placed in front of them with absolutely no explanation or apology. The troubles they had getting any kind of acceptable food cast a pall on our table.

After the first meal, I asked Ruth if she wanted me to make different seating arrangements so that we wouldn't get caught up in this unpleasantness. She emphatically said that we were going to stay at that table. Ruth was livid at their treatment and she wanted to remain at the table and try to help this couple. She did not interfere directly, but she did talk to the woman, who, in turn, spoke in a foreign language to her husband. Ruth tried to make sure that they got something decent to eat every night. Quite a few nights it was poached eggs and bread and butter. She had me speak to the maitre d' in an effort to help them. I was glad to, and I did, but it made no difference. To make a bad situation even worse, the other two couples at our table appeared to enjoy the plight of this hapless couple. Eating on board our ship, at our table, was not a pleasant past time.

That was the only irritant in an otherwise magnificent trip. My own enjoyment, plus Ruth's gratitude for going where she had longed to go for years, made me much richer than the cost of the trip. Both of us were glad that we took the trip.

Within two weeks after our return, Ruth's mother died. We had stayed with her constantly when we got home, but she was in a coma when we got back and didn't recognize us or respond to our conversations. After her mother passed away, Ruth and her brother inherited a lot of money. Ironically, when for the first time in her adult life she would not have to worry about finances, she already was out of the rain under a financial umbrella.

Her mother's death also began to cool the resentment that had smoldered within Ruth. The hurt that she had felt and carried for years would begin to evaporate and lessen.

After all the details of her mother's death had been attended to, Ruth began to press me for more specifics about my family's whereabouts. She found a small, hinged picture frame that contained a picture of my mother and a picture of my father. It was in a box in the cellar along with some of my other possessions. She brought the picture upstairs and put it on her bureau. She often asked why I had no contact with my family and why I did not know where my family was. I told her the truth, I really did not know why I had lost contact with them. We had all just drifted apart. Ruth did not like that answer and she told me so. She told me to try to find my family.

I did work back through the Masons to find out that both my father and mother had died.

That saddened Ruth. I honestly think that she wanted to meet my parents. I wished that she had, she would have loved them and they would have loved her. After seeing how my daughters had responded to Ruth I was sure that love of her was part of the Carp family DNA.

# FALL

The human life cycle follows a strange and wonderful pattern. Each of us enters the world alone and each of us departs alone. Yet, while we are here, we reach towards one another constantly searching for reassurance, companionship, and love. We employ every possible association we can to build these bonds of togetherness. Each of us will use family, religion, race, work, geography, and school as a basis to cling to one another. The list is endless as each of us tries to establish as many of these relationships as he or she can. And of all of these bonds, the strongest, the most noble, is the bond of love. The need for love and respect is deeply rooted within each of us. Without love, we are each diminished to a lesser species of animal.

For me, love was both the balm that eased the pain of life and the nectar that sweetened the joy of life. I always believed that the love between a husband and wife was the sweetest and most satisfying emotion that two humans could ever experience. Certainly part of the foundtion of marital love is sex and the need for sex, but marital love is a more complex feeling than just a sexual urge.

Certainly Ruth and I indulged in sex. For us, it was as natural as our appetites for food and drink. It was just another avenue to express our feelings for one another. We knew that, by itself, sex does not nourish the emotional needs of humans. It is marvelous but, above the steaming passion of the physical act and the wild, joyous orgasm of sex, there is a deeper sentiment.

There is a mysterious force, almost like the pull of a magnetic field, which draws true lovers together. It cannot be defined, or measured, or photographed, but it is there. It radiates from the bodies and the souls of the man and woman intertwined with each other. Together, they generate their own private force field. For those fortunate enough to savor this kind of love it is the most wondrous emotion in the world.

That was the way it was between Ruth and me. We thought of our love as powerful as the energy that has kept the entire universe revolving for millions of years. Something that neither of us tried to define, or explain, but something that we could, and did, fully enjoy. Life was sweet and beautiful.

I don't know why it had to change.

\*\*\*

It seems almost humorous now, but the trip to

Alaska was so beautiful and enjoyable that, after we returned, Ruth began to question her decision to continue working. The money she had inherited from her mother was immediately consolidated with her other assets and she did not change her spending habits. With her inheritance she now had a large money reserve. She invested it all and went, as she said, "From being very cheap, to being very frugal."

It was not her inheritance that changed her mind about working. It became obvious to her that her job prevented us from traveling abroad and she started to consider retirement. After we were together a year and a half, she finally made the decision to stop working.

During the time she was deciding what to do, Ruth and I took no overseas trips. We did whatever we wanted whenever we wanted; we just did it on this continent. We went to a Monet exhibit in Chicago; we toured Key West, The Outer Banks, and Charleston. We went to Toronto to see Showboat. We had fun deciding and planning each of our undertakings and then we enjoyed the adventure itself; but we both knew that our greatest pleasure came from the fact that we were doing it together.

After Ruth did retire, we partook of our daily life with just as much gusto as if each day was a special event. If we were going shopping, and we decided the day was too nice to spend in a grocery store, we would get sandwiches at Zingerman's Deli and go to Gallup Park or we would go to Depot Town and spend a leisurely afternoon drinking coffee at an outside table. If we were making breakfast and we decided to go out to eat, we would turn off the stove and head for the nearest restaurant. If we were running errands and one of us decided that we were horny, we would go home and head for the bedroom. After that we would start out again, laughing at ourselves for being geezer goats. Our long-range plans were based on a time period of one day and our days were scented with the sachet of togetherness.

In the fall of 1995, we received a brochure from the University of Michigan Alumni Office giving details of a tour of Costa Rica in February. Although Ruth enjoyed winter weather, by the time February came I was sure that she would be happy to escape to a sunnier climate. I suggested the trip as a celebration of our third wedding anniversary. After what now had become only a pro forma question, "Can we afford it?" Ruth was delighted at the idea.

As soon as we had paid for the trip, the Alumni Office began bombarding us with pamphlets and books about Costa Rica. We read as much about the country as we could, we scheduled all types of inoculations, and we made all of the other necessary preparations for our departure.

In February we flew first to Houston, and then to the capitol of Costa Rica, San Jose, in commercial jets. After touring San Jose, we flew in a small, single engine propeller plane to Golfito, a port near Panama on the western coast of Costa Rica. There, we boarded a small boat for a three-day cruise northward up the coast.

The minute we entered our tiny cabin we both realized that we were bigger than the space that we had been allotted. The two bunks were attached to the walls on either side of the cabin and set close to the floor. The distance between them was so narrow that we could not get between the bunks without turning sideways and sidling between them. They were neither wide enough nor long enough for us; if we lay straight, the calves of our legs and our feet would hang over the mattress. I spoke first. "Look at these bunks. Terrible! Look at how narrow and short they are. At my age, I don't think I am limber enough to be a contortionist. My guess is that there won't be much screwing going on in this cabin."

Ruth giggled, "Well, I was thinking of pulling you into that tiny shower space. But the walls are so thin that it would be like doing it between two sheets of toilet paper. I guess that I'll have to agree with you, we are not going to be doing it on board this boat." She sighed, "Oh well, let's hope that the food is good."

And it was. The meals were delicious with fresh fruits and vegetables tastefully seasoned and served with elegant cuts of meat or freshly caught fish. We left the boat every day and took long nature walks along the shore. The strange and colorful tropical plants, animals and birds that we glimpsed amazed us. We always returned to our boat tired but pleased. Costa Rica has so much exotic beauty, that at night, when we each retired to our own small bunk, it seemed almost unimportant that we couldn't snuggle.

On one of our tours, we were holding hands and walking along the seashore at Manuel Antonio National Park. We were way behind the other passengers so that no one could hear us, when Ruth said to me, "Honey, for some reason I have always wanted to do it on the sand, right down beside the ocean."

I asked, "Why is that Ladybug? The crabs would certainly bite you, and the sand would chafe your ass."

"Boy, are you ever romantic. It may be absolutely no fun; I just have always wanted to try it."

I said, "In that case, I have just decided to

be romantic. How about right now?"

"Jay, you are not being romantic, you are being impossible. I never said I wanted an audience while we did it."

"Ladybug, that's true. You certainly didn't mention onlookers and there does not seem to be much privacy on this tour. My guess is that we probably won't be doing it in Costa Rica, either on or off the boat." That matter was settled once again, so we continued looking at the flora and fauna.

Our boat trip ended at the port town of Puntarenas, just over midway up the west coast. We were taken by bus to Sarchi, where we spent some time at their farmer's market, a joyous festival of food and color. Every truck was outfitted with its own brightly colored canopy and there were abundant supplies of fresh fish, fruits, and vegetables. It was much larger than the Ann Arbor farmer's market that we were used to, but the relaxed, happy, atmosphere was exactly the same. We were reluctant to leave and inadvertently lingered so long that the tour director had to come and find us. We boarded the bus then and continued on to San Carlos. There, checking in at our resort, we were pleased to find that our room was spacious, clean and attractive. Ruth went directly over to the windows and stood looking out at the scenery. I joined her and we could see nothing but heavy foliage. The hotel was built at the top of a steep hill and there were no buildings in sight. Looking directly down from the windows, I could see nothing but foliage. We both concluded that we were together in our room and that we were alone in our tropical rain forest.

Ruth smiled and asked, "Shall we make up for what we didn't do on the beach at Manuel Antonio?"

We both moved to the bed and started to make love. Very slowly at first, which is the way Ruth enjoyed it, building heat and passion over a long period.

"Honey," Ruth sighed, "Please don't touch my left boob; it is a little painful and sensitive." She always preferred me to massage her right side. I felt sorry for her left boob and I always tried to give it equal treatment, as both of them were a joy to me.

"I am sorry, Ladybug, I did not mean to hurt you."

"Honey, you are gentle. It is just that my left boob is bothering me a little." I tried to be very careful.

Afterwards, we held each other and started a coo and cluck session. At that moment, we saw the faces of a man and woman as they passed by our windows, talking to each other. I don't think they looked into our room, but after they had gone by, I stole a glance at Ruth's face. She was red with embarrassment. She laughed, and said, "In flagrante delicto. You really did want an audience, didn't you?"

"Hell no, I didn't. I don't know where they came from." I jumped out of bed and pulled the curtains together. Later, we walked hand in hand in to the back of the hotel and found a narrow path constructed along the base and all but hidden by the dense foliage. Ruth, looking into our room and finding a clear view of the bed, turned to me and declared that she was never going to do it with me again. I found out the next day that she had changed her mind; what she had really meant was that she was never going to do it again unless the curtains were drawn and the windows were shut.

The remainder of the trip was as exciting as the first half. We saw both an active and a dormant volcano, wondrous spectacles that were new to both of us. We briefly crossed the border into Nicaragua. I am sure that the border crossing was done solely to give us gringo touristas a thrill. Wherever we went, the scenery was magnificent and the food was delicious. We saw things that neither of us had ever seen before and we were delighted with our Costa Rican adventure.

## The Gift of Ruth

\*\*\*

Upon our return, in March of 1996, we quickly went back to our previous routine with one exception. Now that she was retired, Ruth decided to take on more volunteer work for some of the local charities. She had always felt strongly about giving something back to her community. Ruth wanted to help the less fortunate and try to make Ypsilanti a better place. I joined her in doing volunteer work because I shared her convictions.

She selected the activities and we volunteered together. We worked at the polls during elections, and we patrolled for the neighborhood watch association. After our return from Cost Rica, we added volunteering to work for Meals on Wheels twice a month to our activities. Because Ruth had a difficult time saying no to people, she occasionally got stuck with jobs that she really didn't want. Despite great reluctance, she had once agreed to solicit donations from all of the neighbors on our street for one of the national charities. Ruth was asked to write to each of her neighbors and ask them to mail money to her; she would then forward their donations to the charity. Ruth didn't know many of the neighbors personally and she thought she was embarrassing them by writing for money. In turn, she thought that they would embarrass her by not giving any money. She was right. She got absolutely no replies and she felt so bad mailing in only her own donation that she sent the charity a much larger check than she had planned. After that incident, she never undertook the job of writing notes to her neighbors for any charity, no matter how many times she was asked. She just didn't want to go through that experience again.

My own personal preference would have been to work with illiterate people, one on one, trying to teach them to read. I would have enjoyed that. But that would have meant a long-term commitment and it would have interfered with our travel plans. Since I wouldn't be able to stay with it, I chose not to start it.

We also saw a great deal of Dottie and Dick. As couples, we had both signed up for a promotion sponsored by The Cancer Society. For a yearly pledge we were given coupons to a different restaurant each month for six months, and each couple got the least expensive of their two entrées free. The individual restaurants were some of the finest in this area. Unfortunately, because the four of us indulged in before-dinner drinks, hors d'oeuvres, coffee, and dessert, we never saved any money, but we did have one hell of a good time.

We alternated hosting duties at either one of our homes. We would have a few drinks, go to the restaurant of the month and have an excellent meal, and then come back to the host's home and drink black Russians. We seldom broke up before two or three in the morning and the next day was a complete was a complete waste.

\*\*\*

Shortly after we got home from Costa Rica, Ruth made an appointment to see her primary doctor. She had always maintained schedules for mammograms, dental, and medical checkups and she never skipped or delayed any of her appointments. She was conscientious about keeping good health habits to the point that she had stopped smoking years before I returned.

She was having no physical problems aside from the sensitivity in her left breast. Her doctor examined her, checking her breast at Ruth's urging, and he found nothing at all. After the exam, Ruth was furious. She was angry with the doctor for hurting her during the exam and she was also upset that he found nothing. Ruth was worried that the unexplained pain might mean cancer so she made an appointment to see a surgeon.

Looking back, I have been trying to figure out when the web of death started to be woven around Ruth. By the time that the symptoms of her cancer did appear, it was already too late to stop what happened to Ruth. After her death, I went through our 1996 appointment book, checking her appointments. There were no medical meetings listed from March 6, when we returned from Costa Rica, until the April 11 appointment with her primary doctor. She did not see her surgeon, Dr. Martin, until June 11. She had gone to see him several times before and he had examined her and had found nothing suspicious. Ruth must have been seeing him at least since 1995, but Ruth threw out the calendar on which she wrote in her appointments, so I don't know any of those dates.

When Ruth did go to Dr. Martin, in June, he saw something about her left breast that gave him concern. He noticed either a thickening of the skin, or a discoloration of her nipple. Whatever he saw, it was a change. I had gone with Ruth, just to keep her company, and after he examined Ruth, Dr. Martin called me in for a conference. He told us he wanted a biopsy taken, on Ruth's left breast, as soon as possible. July 3rd. was the first date available, so that was the date chosen.

The Fourth of July had always been one of

Ruth's favorite holidays. What made it so special for her were the fireworks displays and the family picnics where she would spend the entire day with her three daughters and all of her grandchildren.

She was almost childlike in her love of fireworks. Every year, we went early to find a spot with a good view to watch the fireworks display at Ford Lake, just down the street from us. Ruth would Ooh, and Aah, as the bright colors filled the night sky with stunning bursts of oranges, reds, blues, yellows, pinks, and greens. She and I had even discussed going with Dottie and Dick and renting motel rooms overnight in Detroit so we could see the fireworks display held alongside the Detroit River, but we never did go. One of Ruth's fondest memories of our visit to Epcot Center was watching the fireworks every night while we were there.

Once the date for the biopsy was established, we knew that our Fourth of July celebration would be different than it had been in previous years. I wasn't sure that Ruth would want to sit in one place for hours the day after her biopsy. We would not be able to take our folding chairs at dusk, and wait by the lake until ten or eleven at night just to be sure we had a good place to see the fireworks. Both of us were apprehensive.

The Marriott motel, located on the other side of Ford Lake from where we lived, solved the problem by advertising a "Fourth of July Special." They would provide a room overlooking the lake, from where we could watch the fireworks, and also serve their guests a full breakfast the next morning.

When I suggested this idea to Ruth, she, at first, demurred. She did not know how she would feel the day after her outpatient surgery, the cost would be too expensive, and we might not get a good view of the fireworks. She came up with a list of all the reasons we shouldn't rent the room. After thinking about it though, she began to like the idea. She then suggested that her daughters, and all her grandchildren, could come up to the room, join us, and watch the fireworks.

I emphatically told Ruth something I rarely said to her. I said, "No."

I had never before denied her anything regarding her children or grandchildren. But Ruth was my major concern and I thought a hotel room, filled with seven or eight adults who were heavy smokers, and five or six active grandchildren, would be too much for her. When I explained that to her, I said that the room was not for them, they could follow the same routine they had followed for years. The room was only meant for us so that we could see the fireworks. We talked about it for a while, and she eventually agreed with me.

All things considered, the Fourth of July week turned out well. Ruth had her biopsy at 7:00 AM on Wednesday. She was a little woozy, and had some pain, but not enough of either to prevent her from trying to enjoy the holiday festivities. We checked into the Marriott early in the afternoon and watched the fireworks that evening. Looking at them, through a window in an air-conditioned room, was not as much fun as seeing them out of doors. On the other hand, Ruth would not have been comfortable sitting in a lawn chair for hours.

The next morning, Thursday, I drove home, fed Ruth's two cats, Bonnie and Clyde, and then returned in time to have breakfast with Ruth. That evening, we went to see The Capitol Steps, who were appearing at the U of M Power Center. Friday, Saturday, and Sunday, we were at home in our own bed. Each morning we cooed and clucked an extra long time, not getting up until well after 8:00 A.M. We just talked and held each other. Neither of us thought about sex. Both of us could not forget the snippet of tissue that had been cut out of Ruth's breast. What we were doing was reaffirming our commitment to one another without any direct statements.

*Jay Carp*

This year, the family Fourth of July picnic was held on Sunday. For many years, Ruth had been a member in a swimming club that was associated with a private lake located on a farm. The man who owned the farm sold memberships and the members, along with the few homeowners whose property fronted the lake on the other side, were the only people permitted to swim there. It was a pleasant, clean place to go swimming in the summer time. When they were young, Ruth had taken her three daughters to the lake almost every weekend during the summers. Christie and Tracy had become members of the club after they started raising their own families, and Robin came on an occasional basis. The lake, and the family gatherings held there, were an important part of all of their lives.

I enjoyed the outings as much as Ruth and her girls did. Her girls were pleased that I treated them as my own and they were happy that I did not try to change any of their rules or customs. They often told me that their mother's disposition had definitely improved after I came back into her life. I liked her daughters, I liked her daughter's children, and I liked her daughter's husbands. What I did not enjoy was the week of preparation that took place before the picnic. Like any other event that included her daughters, there would be endless phone calls among the four of them to discuss who was going to bring what, what day to hold the outing, and what to do in case of rain. They would decide on these matters, hang up the phone, and, minutes later, think of something else, and immediately call each other back. Finally, when all was said and done, each would do the same things, bring the same things, and arrive at the same times as they had done every previous year. I studiously avoided getting involved in this farce as much as I possibly could.

Ruth was determined that we attend the picnic, and I was all for it. I asked her daughters that their procedures be changed so that Ruth would not be responsible for making the cole slaw, which she traditionally brought. The girls readily agreed, but convincing Ruth was a little harder. After a while, she reluctantly conceded.

We went to the picnic a little later, and we left a little earlier, than we normally would. And it was a happy occasion. Robin, Christie, and Tracy, along with Christie's and Tracy's husbands, and all six of the grandchildren were there. They were grouped around Ruth stuffing-her with food, conversation, and family memories. Everyone enjoyed the good weather and each other's company. On the way home, Ruth kept patting my arm and thanking me for the nice weekend and for accepting her family without any reservations. I was touched. I covered it up by telling her that I had three daughters and she had three daughters and when you added them together the total sum was six individual pains in the ass. She knew that, because they were her daughters, I would love them exactly as I loved my daughters.

We cuddled, cooed and clucked extra long that Sunday night and Monday morning. Both of us had concerns about the future, so we stayed with the present.

***

About ten o'clock on the Monday following the Fourth of July weekend we got the answer we didn't want to the question we hadn't asked. Ruth got a phone call telling her that her scheduled appointment to see Dr. Martin on Thursday, July 11, was cancelled and that an appointment to see an oncologist was being set up for Wednesday, July 10. Ruth had just stepped onto the merry-goround that was going to spin her away from me forever. One year and three days after that first appointment she would be gone.

That Wednesday we met her oncologist, Dr. Elinor Curry. She came into the room where we were waiting, a slim, young looking woman.

She introduced herself, asked us both a few personal questions, and then, in a professional but sympathetic manner, she explained the results of the biopsy. We had already surmised that it was cancer. Dr. Curry asked Ruth if she wanted to hear the details. She explained that many of her patients were afraid to be told anything, and if Ruth did not wish to hear more she should make her wishes known. Ruth of course, wanted to hear all of the information. Being honest and frank herself, Ruth insisted on the same from her doctor.

We were inundated with detail after detail. I was overwhelmed and I suspect that Ruth was as well; however, I am sure that she understood a lot more of the information than I did. Basically, the doctor told us that the cancer was so large that they were going to start chemotherapy immediately to try to reduce it. They would then remove the cancer by surgery, followed by more chemotherapy. After all the chemotherapy treatments were finished, there would be a series of radiation treatments.

During our long discussion, Dr. Curry was absolutely straightforward and solemn as she had important personal news to impart and none of it was good news. She was careful not to raise false hopes, but neither did she want to encourage despair. Dr. Curry was a human being caught up in an inhuman job. She explained that the chemotherapy treatments would cause Ruth to lose her hair, and that she could be tired, or nauseous, or weak. It was impossible to predict Ruth's exact symptoms because each individual reacted differently to the strong chemicals that were pumped through their body.

It seemed that the doctor spoke patiently to both of us for hours. Ruth and I were numb; we were beyond grief. How could such a terrible thing have happened to us? I sat there, hearing words, listening hard to all of this, but not really comprehending. I drifted away from the conversation and kept thinking, "Why should this happen to Ruth? What has she done to deserve this?" I came back when Dr. Curry was explaining to Ruth that her attitude towards her treatment would be very important. It was at this point that Ruth asked the doctor, point blank, what her chances of beating the cancer were.

Responding in very carefully measured words the doctor was neither optimistic nor pessimistic. She told us that every cancer was different, every patient was different, and that each patient's response was different. Results might not be certain until years after the treatment. A basic rule of thumb, though, would be to hope for a five-year rescission rate; if the cancer didn't reappear within that time, the treatments had been successful.

Then came the task of scheduling. The first chemotherapy treatment was set up for July 18th, eight days after our appointment with Dr. Curry. In the meantime, there were other tests that needed to be done before the first chemo treatment began. Appointments for a bone scan, mammograms and ultrasounds, and something called a Muga, were scheduled before we left the doctor's office.

When we got back to the car, Ruth squeezed my hand tightly, and said, in an angry tone of voice, "Son of a bitch, I told them that I had breast cancer, and they wouldn't believe me. Shit, why should this happen now? After all these years, I finally find someone I love. I am so happy, and then I get tagged with breast cancer. Shit." She thought for a moment and added, "Oh well, at least I will get to pick out the color for my new hair when I get a wig."

We drove from St. Joseph Mercy Hospital back to our house and Ruth called her daughters who were anxious to hear what she had found out. She talked to each one patiently, telling them everything that we had learned. Each one of them broke down upon hearing that she had cancer and she told them to stop crying and calm themselves. Of course they were upset, but Ruth told them that there was a good chance that the treatments could get all of the cancer and that she could live a long life. She said that she wanted them to think positively and act positively; that was the only way she could beat her cancer.

That afternoon and evening, we made, and received a lot of phone calls. I called each of my daughters and told them about Ruth. They took the news the same way Ruth's daughters did; they broke down. I comforted them the same way that Ruth had comforted her daughters.

She and I talked about what was facing each of us. We went over all the possibilities and Ruth never tried to sugarcoat what might happen. It was a gloomy time. She certainly was brave. In no uncertain terms Ruth told me that we both had to have a positive attitude and assume that she would live another twenty five years. She refused to have our friends and family feeling sorry for us. She and I were to continue calmly and enjoy what we could.

From that day forward, Ruth's medical schedule dictated what our other plans were to be. On the day that Ruth's first chemo treatment was now scheduled, we had made previous plans to go into Detroit with Dottie and Dick. We were supposed to eat supper at the Rattlesnake Club, go gambling in Windsor, and stay overnight night in Canada. Ruth called Dottie and changed the date to two days before her treatment. There was no way that Ruth was going to miss being with her friends.

That morning, before we met Dick and Dottie, as we lay in bed, I began to slowly caress Ruth. After a long time, she began to quietly respond, and we both began to get excited. It was our first sex in over a month.

Afterwards, Ruth snuggled against me and said, "Honey, I am sorry. I know it has been a long time since we did it, but I just have not been in the mood."

"Hush, Ladybug, you do not owe me any apologies. With everything that is happening I can understand."

She raised up in bed to look at me. "Maybe," she said, "But I surely do enjoy it when I am in the mood. Do you think that going through chemo, and radiation, and losing my boob will change my attitude, and that I will never get horny again?"

"Wife, after all the treatments are finished, I would be very surprised if you stopped getting horny. I don't think we will ever be doing it on a beach, but I do think that we will be doing it."

And we did, the very next morning in our motel in Windsor. When we got back to our house, Ruth had her grandson, Ritchie, come over with his barber's clippers and crop her hair. She said that, if her hair had to fall out, she did not want it clogging up the drains.

The next day, Ruth started her chemo treatments. The process surprised both of us and I really don't know why we should have been surprised. Until we arrived at the hospital, neither of us had any idea of how patients were treated, or how chemotherapy was administered. The attention given to each patient astonished us. The staff showered each patient with respect and comfort as they went about their essential task of pouring chemicals into these sick bodies. To ease the shock of this traumatic experience, great care was given in explaining to Ruth and me what would happen and what she should expect.

Lew, the nurse assigned to take care of Ruth met us in the waiting room; he would administer the chemo treatments after talking with us. He introduced himself, brought us into a small consultation room, and described what to expect both with the treatments themselves and any possible side effects. Lew told us that, behind the scenes, a great deal of thought is put into the dosage for each patient. The chemicals injected into the patient's body are powerful and harsh and they can destroy the good as well the bad. Because of that, the types of drugs and the doses are decided upon by a group of experts.

The treatment is brutal, so the blood work of the patient is closely monitored to make sure that the patient can tolerate the next treatment. Susceptibility to colds and flu are a particular concern. Ruth's blood would be drawn before all treatments to insure that her red cells and her white cells were within acceptable limits.

After answering all of our questions, Lew took us into the treatment room. It was not at all what I had envisioned, there were no beds. Instead, There were about twenty reclining chairs close to each other and the chairs that held patients had drip poles beside the chair. The drip poles had plastic bags of chemical and saline solutions slung from them and the contents were fed into the patient's veins through plastic tubing leading to a needle in the patient's arm. The room looked cluttered. To me, it seemed like a quiet battlefield where each patient was slowly and silently fighting to stay alive.

Lew was attentive as he walked us through the treatment room and got Ruth situated in one of the chairs. He explained the entire procedure to us, only interrupting his discussion while he administered medications or encouraged another of his patients.

After Lew finished his explanations, he pierced her vein, started the chemicals flowing into her body, and then he left. He came back at least every five or ten minutes to see how she was doing and to reassure her. Ruth was grateful to Lew for his concern and, after a few visits, she referred to him as her "Floor Angel."

Our final surprise was the attitude of everyone in that room, both the patients and the staff. The possibility of death sifts the churlishness out of people. There was a pleasant, polite, and friendly air in the treatment room. If you didn't wish to speak, you were left alone; if you wanted conversation you could easily find someone willing to talk. The treatment room was a serene place, like a house of worship.

Ruth was scheduled for three chemo treatments, one month apart, before her partial mastectomy. Lew told her to be alert for possible side effects and to call him immediately if she had any questions. He said that it was important to get a full dosage of chemicals into her body as quickly as possible to fight her cancer. He did not want to delay the treatments, and that was why he encouraged her to call if she had any questions. Lew was a good nurse and he took his job of trying to help people very seriously.

Ruth did have reactions to the chemotherapy treatments. A pattern developed after each one. She would feel sick to her stomach the first two weeks The week after that she would feel pretty good, and her appetite would begin to return and she could taste her food; the last week and until her next treatment, she would be close to feeling normal. Throughout the course of the chemotherapy treatments, she did feel weak and she did tire easily; but she fought against all of these symptoms. She wanted to feel better, so she tried to overcome anything that stood in her way. Ruth was a fighter.

The week before she was scheduled to receive her second chemo treatment, I noticed a change in Ruth's attitude. In our coo and clucks she would not say much and she would cling to me tightly, like a strand of seaweed on dry skin. I felt for her, but I said nothing. I knew that whatever was bothering Ruth would surface when she was ready and not before. So, I held her and waited.

The morning before her treatment she finally spoke up. "I had a friend who had cancer and she had to have both of her boobs removed. Her son of a bitch of a bastard husband divorced her less than a year after her surgery."

I felt so foolish. We had talked about everything else associated with her cancer, but we had never discussed her mastectomy. I knew that she was afraid of losing her breast and I had assumed that was why we hadn't talked about it before.

"Ladybug, look at me," I said. When we

were face to face, I kissed her, and continued, "You need to understand that you are stuck with me. You are going to lose a breast you might lose two. Whatever you lose, you will not lose me. 'For better or for worse,' is what we pledged to each other, and 'For better or for worse' is the way it is going to be. I am where I want to be, with you, and I am not leaving."

"Oh Honey, how can you say that? They are going to cut off my left boob and I won't be a pretty woman anymore."

I did not answer for a while. She was deeply concerned, and I wanted to reassure her. Finally, I asked, "Ruth, would you leave me if I had to have either my balls or my pecker chopped off?"

"Why no, of course I wouldn't leave you. It would change things, but not my love. Men are different though, they want their women to have two boobs."

"Wife, I can't vouch for all men, I can only talk as your husband. Right now, you have all the standard equipment that other women have. That is going to change, but so what? You are my wife. I want you as my wife and you will always be my wife.

"Sure, I will miss your boobie, the same way you would miss any of my equipment if it were lopped off. Boobies are fine, but I have something more important. I have you, and that is more than I ever hoped for. I don't want to leave; I can't leave; I won't leave. You are stuck with me and I could not be happier."

Ruth lay quietly by my side a long time. Finally, she stirred a little and kissed me on the cheek. "Thank you, Honey," she said. "I really needed that. I absolutely adore you. Not only that, but your speech made me horny. It is entirely your fault, so you had better do something about it."

***

It was sometime between her second and third chemo treatment that Ruth received a message asking her to make an appointment to see Dr. Karen Barnett. Dr. Barnett was to be her radiation oncologist. Even though it was now August, and Ruth would not start her radiation treatments until next January, Dr. Barnett made a practice of meeting her patients as soon as possible. I drove Ruth over to the hospital for her first appointment with Dr. Barnett, but I did not meet her at that time. When Ruth came out of her office, she told me that she liked her both as a physician and as a person. She said that Dr. Barnett was very upbeat in her attitude and had recommended that Ruth try vitamins to build up Ruth's immune system. They were very expensive so Ruth told Dr. Barnett that she would have to check with me.

"Ruth why did you even bother telling Dr. Barnett you would have to check with me? Screw the damn expense. If there is the slightest chance that those pills will help, get them. The cost is none of your business. Please order them."

"I told Dr. Barnett that you would say that. She is going to go ahead and order me the health and vitamin pills. The order will take a while, but I am to start taking them as soon as they arrive.

"Incidentally, you are supposed to come with me on my next visit. Dr. Barnett always schedules at least one family visit early so that she can meet the family and explain her procedures. I think you'll be impressed with her."

Ruth was correct, when I did meet Dr. Barnett I was impressed. She was a tall, attractive woman with a lot of energy and a lot of interests besides medicine. She herself had had surgery at St. Joseph's, a few years back, and, as a patient, she detested the hospital system. When she returned to work as a doctor, she insisted on making reforms that made the hospital procedures much more patient friendly.

She explained to us why radiation was

deemed necessary and how it would be done. She told us what the side effects might be and what could be done to help the patient. She also said that recovery from the side effects would take about five or six months after the last radiation treatment.

Dr. Barnett told Ruth that a special cradle would have to be made to hold Ruth's body in the same precise position during each of the radiation treatments. A committee that included herself, a physicist, a nurse, and a machine technician would determine the radiation dosage, and oversee the administration of the radiation.

Dr. Barnett went through all of this slowly, so that we could ask questions if we thought of them. After our indoctrination was finished, I left so that the doctor could conduct her personal examination of Ruth.

As Ruth and I were walking through the parking lot after the examination, she casually said, "Dr. Barnett said that she takes the same health and vitamins pills that she is recommending for me. She went through the manufacturing facility in California to satisfy herself of their purity. I will be getting a shipment of pills, once a month and the billing will automatically appear on our Visa card statement. They are very expensive. Do you still think it is all right, Honey?"

"Ladybug, don't even bother to ask. You are a bona fide pain in the ass. I am for anything that has a chance of helping. Let's change the subject. Do you feel able to go with me tomorrow on our neighborhood watch patrol?"

Throughout all of her medical appointments for blood work, exams, x-rays, and chemo treatments, Ruth had attempted to maintain as normal a life as she could. She was trying very hard to meet her social obligations and enjoy her personal commitments. We had just returned from Trumansberg, New York, where we had visited Edward, and his wife, Joan. On the way, we had made it a point to stay overnight in Lockport and see the Erie Canal. We were fascinated by the old locks, and enjoyed watching the boats go through the modern locks. Ruth had a good time, but she was worn out when we arrived home. I wanted to make sure that she did not over extend herself, she needed a lot of rest.

As part of our commitment to patrol the neighborhood, we were scheduled to drive around for a two-hour shift. All that we had to do was ride around the neighborhood and note anything unusual in our logbook, never leaving our vehicle or confronting anyone. We were just to observe. Ruth enjoyed patrolling, and we would chat while I drove. However, if she did not feel up to it, I could do it by myself.

"Of course I can do it and I will," Ruth said. "There is no excuse not to."

Two weeks after Ruth saw Dr. Barnett she had her third chemo treatment. After that, the following weeks were taken up with more medical exams and doctor's appointments in preparation for her surgery. On the thirtieth of August Ruth went into St. Joseph Mercy Hospital and had a modified radical mastectomy. Two days later she was forced to leave the hospital with a catheter sticking out of her.

She had wanted to stay in the hospital an extra day because she did not feel well either physically or mentally. She had hoped for just one more day to try to reconcile herself to the fact that she hurt and that her body had been disfigured. She needed time to face her new reality.

However that was not to be. Mastectomies are allowed to stay in the hospital for two days. There could be no extenuating circumstances. That was the dictate of The Gods of The Hospitals, our insurance companies.

I was livid with rage when Ruth was pushed out of the door. Never mind the traumas and the emotions of the patients; the bean counters determine the length of your stay. Never mind the doctor and patient relationship; cost analysis determines when you will vacate your hospital bed. Whatever happened to compassion in this system? Whatever happened to loving care? Would it have hurt them to grant another twenty-four hours to a woman who was truly physically and mentally sick? I spit on a system that uses cost to force a dying woman out of her hospital bed. I took that as a personal insult to Ruth.

And so Ruth came home, a day earlier than she wanted, not feeling well physically, and mourning the loss of her left breast. She did her best to fight the pain and the depression of disfigurement but it was hard for her. For a week her body hurt her badly and her incision seeped through the bandages. She would go into the bathroom and shut the door when she changed dressings; she did not want me to see her.

After about ten days the pain finally began to subside and the fluids stopped seeping. Ruth began to feel better physically, and she tried to resume her activities. We went for flu shots, and, towards the end of October, we went away for a quiet weekend at a bed and breakfast, near the Upper Peninsula. We had selected the weekend just before her fourth chemo treatment as the weekend to go away.

It was odd how our lives had changed and how quickly we had adapted. Prior to Ruth's cancer, the calendar was the metronome that beat the rhythm of what we did. Now, her chemo treatments shaped the boundaries of all our other activities.

The pace quickened after Ruth's surgery and her remaining chemo treatments were given on a different schedule; she now received them approximately every three weeks. As we had with the monthly treatments, we fitted everything else around them.

The first two weeks after the treatment, we would schedule as little as possible so that Ruth could recover from the side effects. As soon as she felt better, we would do things together. Luncheons at good restaurants, movies we both wanted to see, concerts, the farmer's market, whatever was available when we were ready was fine with us. I was grateful just to see Ruth recover from the effects of the chemicals.

The third week was the time we selected for our dinner dates with Dottie and Dick and community activities such as Meals on Wheels and neighborhood watch patrols. Ruth even worked as an election official, although she did not stay the entire fourteen hours that the polls were open.

From October through early December of 1996, Ruth had three more chemo treatments and that was the end of them. Her radiation therapy was scheduled to start early in January of 1997. That gave us almost a whole month free of any kind of medical appointments; the pause couldn't have come at a better time.

***

Around the middle of December, as Ruth began to realize that the chemo treatments were over and that Christmas was coming, she started to feel more of the holiday spirit. She had always enjoyed the Christmas season and this year was no exception. She relished agonizing over the sweaters, skirts, and clothing that she bought for her daughters and granddaughters, complaining that they would not like the colors, that the sizes would be wrong, and that almost everything would have to be exchanged. To her, the shopping, the selecting, and even the gift returning on the day after Christmas were integral parts of the holiday activities. Unlike the rest of the year, she kept the receipts carefully isolated until after Christmas Day, when she would talk to her daughters and find out what items of clothing would have to be exchanged.

Depending on her mood, Ruth either agreed, or disagreed, with my approach to Christmas. I was tired of the heavy handed commercialism that was tarnishing the spirit of the holiday, especially the pressures put on parents and grandparents to buy toys and junk products for their offspring. To save myself the frustrations of shopping, and to avoid over indulging my grandkids, I gave each of my daughters a check to buy whatever they wanted for themselves, and I bought a savings bond for each of the grandchildren. Although Ruth thought about trying my approach, she told me that her daughters and grandchildren would be disappointed if they received money instead of personal gifts. So, her Christmas shopping continued.

Christmas lights delighted Ruth. She loved to see the light displays at Riverside Park in Ypsilanti and Domino's Farm in Ann Arbor. Every year, we would drive around our own neighborhood two or three times a week looking at the lights and, whenever we went anywhere, Ruth would ask me to detour each time she saw a new display. One night, three years ago, as we were leaving Ann Arbor on Washtenaw Road, she asked me to drive around Tuomy Hills. That was the neighborhood where we had both been living when we first met. There were some beautiful light displays and we drove around slowly, admiring them, and pointing out different features to each other. After that, Ruth added the Austin Avenue light display to her list of things to do for Christmas.

During past Christmas seasons, Ruth had not wanted me to go shopping with her. It took her so long to decide what to buy that she preferred the leisure of solitude. This year was different. Because she tired so easily she was glad to have me accompany her to help her carry her packages and to help her make up her mind.

One afternoon, late in December, after a shopping trip, Ruth was cold, so she decided to take a hot shower. She always would have the bathroom door shut while she showered so that the room would be steamy and warm when she stepped out of the tub. She would dry herself, and then open the door so that the moisture on the mirror could evaporate. After the door was open she would talk to me if she had anything to say. I would answer her, but usually she could not hear me because the door would only be partially open and she would be busy applying powder or makeup. She would call out to me to come to the door and we would continue talking. She would be moving around stark naked while I would be standing still fully clothed. Since her operation, she had never opened the door. She had become very guarded and defensive about her body.

This time, she did call out and ask me to come by the door. When I did, I saw that it was barely ajar, and by looking through the small

265

opening I could just see her backside. I opened the door a few inches wider. As Ruth was talking she turned to the mirror and saw me looking in. After a moment's hesitation, she opened her mouth and put her right hand over her left chest, as if she were going to recite the Pledge of Allegiance. She continued to stare at my image in the mirror.

I opened the door. Ruth turned from the mirror to face me. Challenged, she raised her chin and then slowly lowered her hand to her side while she stared at me. The scar ran horizontally from the middle of her chest to her left armpit. It looked red and angry. My heart leaped in sympathy as I thought how tormented she must be.

I stared at her naked body with no expression on my face. I took the time to look her up and down twice before saying, "Ladybug, you don't seem to have lost much hair from your Hmm-Hmm."

During the time that I looked at her, some ten or fifteen seconds, Ruth watched me intently to see if I was going to flinch or draw back. Her response was loud with fear and anger. "Jay, look at me. Don't you think that I am ugly? Don't you think I am disfigured? A freak? Isn't that what you are thinking?"

I put my hand on her cheek and stroked

her face. I was on the verge of tears as I said, "Ruth, you are not ugly. You are not disfigured. You are not a freak. You are a woman who has had a breast removed and your body shows it.

"Sure there is a scar on the outside. But your heart is still inside and your love is still inside. You are my wife whether with one boob or two. As a matter of fact, the only thing that I am thinking right now is that I am getting horny."

Ruth's face began to work as if she were going to cry, but she fought against that by coming into my arms and squeezing me fiercely to the right side of her body. She murmured, "Oh Jay, I love you so much. I am so glad that you came back to see my mother. Why the Hell didn't you ever call me after we broke up?

"Horny? You are, without a doubt a dirty old man and I am grateful for that. I can't take care of your horniness right now, but there will be a time when I will. Is that all right Honey?"

Just having Ruth begin to feel good about herself again was enough for me.

\*\*\*

Christmas of 1996 was a relatively quiet one. The activities and the hubbub were reduced but not the satisfaction. We had Ruth's daughters and the grandchildren over the night before and we opened all of our exchange presents. The girls brought me over a birthday cake and birthday cards for my birthday on the twenty-fourth.

Ruth and I got up early on Christmas Day and exchanged presents and emptied our stockings. I showered her with presents even though she had made me promise not to spend much on her this Christmas. I surprised her with gift certificates for body massages because she had had a massage once and she thought that it was delightful. I figured that, when her strength began to return, the indulgence would make her feel better.

By far, though, the present that pleased Ruth the most was the birdfeeder I got for her. Sometime after midnight on Christmas Eve, while Ruth slept, I dug a hole in the frozen ground, installed the pole, and placed the feeder on the pole. Then, I filled it with sunflower seeds and put the receipt for the sixty-pound bag of bird feed in her stocking along with some Burger King gift certificates.

After we opened our big presents, we took our stockings off the mantle and went through them. At first Ruth was confused when she found the bird feed receipt, but when she opened the curtains and saw the birdfeeder standing near the window, she was delighted. She spent many hours talking to her "pretty" birds, cardinals, nuthatches, and grosbeaks and asking the "ordinary" birds, swallows, pigeons, and starlings to go away. I wondered why I hadn't put up a feeder years before.

We called my girls and Ruth and I talked to each of them for a long time and wished them a Merry Christmas. The girls were comfortable with Ruth and were glad that she was feeling better.

New Year's Eve was also a quiet celebration. We went out to eat early and then we went to the Ypsilanti Jubilee. It was patterned after Boston's First Night in that it was meant to be a family celebration. The Jubilee is an alcohol free event held downtown in Ypsilanti with all types of entertainment available. Jazz combos, pianists, dulcimer players, and singers give concerts throughout the evening in almost every church and meeting hall. For anyone not interested in music there are storytellers, comedians, and magicians. Shuttle busses circulate throughout the evening to help everyone get to the various events. For the price of one ticket you can rotate through and select whatever kind of entertainment you want. We concentrated on going to the jazz concerts because we both liked jazz.

Ruth and I ended up kissing and wishing each other Happy New Year while dancing to a

big band era orchestra. The midnight that ush-
ered in 1997 started the saddest year of my life.
And it arrived quietly and with so much hope
that Ruth had beaten her cancer.

***

Ruth started her radiation treatments right after the first of the year. Her schedule called for
twenty-seven sessions given daily five times a
week. They were administered at the same location where Ruth had received her chemo treatments, the St. Joseph Cancer Center. When we
arrived, Ruth would go to the dressing room
and don a hospital johnny. She would go to the
specific machine designated for her use that day
and climb into her specially fitted "cradle." The
radiation dosage itself lasted only a few minutes. After that, she would meet me in the lobby
where I would be waiting. The whole procedure
never took more than twenty-five minutes.

While I waited, I would usually watch the
beautiful tropical fish that were swimming in a
huge fish tank in the center of the waiting room. I
would also check their coffee and cookie supply.
If they had any small packages of Lorna Doone
cookies, I would get two packages for Ruth. After we got into the car, I would hand them over
to her and she would smile and thank me.

One morning, as I read a magazine, Lloyd

Carr, the Michigan football coach came in and took a seat. He had been head coach for two years and his record for each year was eight wins and four losses. The alumni expected a much better performance than that and he had been subjected to a lot of questioning and second-guessing. He was by himself and I thought about going over and talking to him but I figured he was probably here with someone who was getting treatments and that he would prefer to be left alone. With that in mind, I just sat there and continued to read my magazine.

This was the second time I had seen him in person. The first had been the evening that his status had been changed from "interim" head coach to head coach. Dottie, Dick, Ruth and I had been eating at a downtown restaurant and, when Dottie saw him, she went over to his table and congratulated him and wished him good luck. When she came back to our table, Dottie couldn't get over the fact that she had talked to the new head coach of the Michigan football team.

When Ruth joined me, after her treatment, I pointed him out to her. As we were looking, a lady wearing a blue baseball cap with a gold M on it came out of the dressing room, and they both left together.

Ruth said, "That must be Lloyd Carr's

mother. I have talked to her a few times and she is a very pleasant woman. I didn't know who she was but the next time I talk to her I am going to ask her if she would get her son to give me an autograph that says, 'To Dottie, from Lloyd Carr'. Boy, wouldn't that knock Dottie's sox off?"

We never saw either Lloyd Carr or his mother at the Cancer Center again, so Dottie never did get her personalized autograph.

The first time I met Dr. Barnett I had asked her when she thought that Ruth would recover from the side effects of the radiation treatments. She answered that, by May or June, Ruth should begin to feel good. With those months in mind, I began to think about a trip for Ruth as a reward for all that she had endured.

In late December, the Alumni Association sent us pamphlets on two trips that they were offering in the May or June time frame. One was a trip to the Greek Isles and the other was a trip to Russia. My first reaction was that Ruth would probably enjoy the trip to Greece more than the trip to Russia. Greece was one of the places we had talked about when we discussed using my frequent flyer miles. I still had over 200,000 miles that I had accrued from the business trips I took before I retired.

When I read the brochures, I thought that

the trip to Greece would be the better of the two for Ruth. The sunshine of Greece would definitely buoy her spirits and that area of the world was supposed to be spectacular. However, when we started asking questions, we found that there was a lot of physical activity involved in taking that particular tour. We would be climbing steep hills to historical sites, riding burros or mules over narrow trails, and walking over uneven ground. These activities made me believe that the trip would be wearing on Ruth.

The Russian tour was much less demanding. We would fly into Moscow, stay there a day or two examining the city, and then go by boat, from Moscow to St. Petersburg. The boat would serve as our hotel throughout the trip, and, although we would do a lot of sightseeing, the activities would not be overly strenuous. We weren't sure which trip we would enjoy more.

On a personal basis, Russia intrigued me. For over twenty years I had worked on the Inter Continental Ballistic Missile system, Minuteman. The sole purpose of Minuteman was to act as a deterrent against a Russian nuclear attack. As a result of the Cold War, the United States had thousands of nuclear warheads aimed at the Soviet Union. I had always wanted to see the country that had provoked so much fear in my own nation. Although I personally considered mismanagement and stupidity to be the biggest threats to world peace, both GTE and the Air Force were constantly reminding me that it really was the Russians.

I had no trouble believing that the Communist government was a brutal dictatorship, however, I did not believe that all of the people living under that evil regime were themselves vicious animals. How could a people produce such beautiful music and dancing if they were bereft of all humanity? If I had learned anything during my life it was that prejudice helps people make dishonest judgements.

My daughter, Cynthia, once told me an interesting story about a trip that she had taken to Russia. In 1978, her husband, Allen, was in the Air Force and assigned to an air base in England. From there, he and Cynthia took a tour of St. Petersburg and Moscow. The evening that they arrived in Moscow, they had tickets to see the Bolshoi Ballet. They got to the theater just as the ballet was beginning and my daughter, who had to go the bathroom, decided she did not want to miss any of the performance. Instead, she found out that the lady's room was two floors above where they were seated and she decided to wait until intermission.

As soon as the first act ended, even before the curtain closed, Cynthia was out of her seat, running for the stairs, and going up the two flights of stairs as fast as she could. When she arrived at the lady's room, she took her place at the end of the line behind ten or twelve other women. There she was, a slightly overweight young lady, panting heavily after she had dashed up the stairs, and hopping from foot to foot because she had to go to the bathroom.

A middle-aged matron just ahead of Cynthia kept turning and looking at her. She must have become concerned because she finally said something in Russian. Cynthia, not understanding what the woman was saying, patted her chest and said slowly, "I am an American. I am sorry, but I do not speak Russian."

The woman nodded and then, in French, she asked Cynthia if she understood that language. Cynthia answered her in fluent French. Speaking French, the woman apologized for asking personal questions, but said she had noticed that Cynthia seemed very distressed. Cynthia answered the lady quickly, and told her a bald faced lie. She said, "Thank you, I am not distressed, but I do need to go the bathroom, and I am pregnant."

The woman again nodded her head, turned and spoke in Russian to the other women who were ahead of both of them. Lo and behold, all the women stepped aside and Cynthia was the next one to use the toilet.

I asked Cynthia if she didn't feel bad about lying to the lady just to get to the head of the line. She told me that she did have some qualms, but only after she had left the bathroom to return to the performance. This story has always appealed to me because of the humanity the Russian woman displayed, and because it shows that not all Russians are bad and not all Americans are good.

Despite my leaning towards the trip to Russia, I kept my preferences to myself. This was Ruth's trip and she should decide where she wanted to go without my trying to influence her. I would be with her, no matter what her choice was, so I couldn't lose either way.

She took a long time before deciding. Her normal reluctance to make any decision before the last minute was part of the delay but there were also other reasons. It had been a cold, dreary, Michigan winter and she had been taking radiation treatments daily. For Ruth, it was a pleasant past time, deciding which trip to take. So she dallied, listing the pros and cons of each trip. Finally, despite her keen desire to go to Greece, she chose the tour of Russia because she knew that it would be less physically demanding. We signed up for it, and we were scheduled to fly to Moscow at the end of May. It gave Ruth something to look forward to while she endured the rest of her radiation treatments.

\*\*\*

As it turned out, Ruth needed something to bolster her spirits. Towards the end of January, the daily dosages of radiation began to burn her skin. The burns were severe enough to stop the treatments before the calculated number of dosages was reached. Dr. Barnett told Ruth that, once the treatment was stopped to allow the skin to heal, the effectiveness of the radiation could not be retained. So, for all practical purposes, her treatments were over. Dr. Barnett also told Ruth that she had actually received the recommended amount of radiation for her cancer. The last few treatments that she was not going to get would have been directed towards the scar tissue on her chest. Those treatments were to be an insurance policy against the cancer returning to the skin area.

All of a sudden, all medical treatments were over and we were left to adjust to the aftermath. The doctors had tried every procedure available to them, surgery, chemicals, and radiation to defeat the malignancy within Ruth's body. There was nothing more that they could do for her. Ruth was left to deal with the aftermath of these severe medical procedures.

She had forced herself to adapt to each change as it occurred. She tried to be positive and played down her weakness and her tiredness. She wore bright colored turbans on her head most of the time unless we went to a fancy restaurant. Then, she would wear her wig, which she absolutely detested. It was a good looking hairpiece and it looked a lot like her natural hair, but Ruth did not think so and she dreaded wearing it.

Her biggest problem, though, was adjusting to her missing breast. She felt that, without it, she was not a woman and she mourned for her lost breast. She was certain that no matter what outfit she wore, and no matter what prosthesis she wore under her clothes, from a rolled up sock to a plastic breast fitted by an expert, everyone could see her disfigurement. It took a long time for her to come to grips with her loss.

During her radiation treatments, and while her burnt skin was healing, Ruth did not want sex. That was not a major concern for me as I could see what she was trying to cope with, so I said nothing and did nothing. My concern was that I wanted Ruth to feel better. I knew that Ruth was not shy and when she was ready she would let me know. I hoped, for her sake as well as my own, that she would feel the need again.

It was a different time for us. Since we couldn't cuddle, our coo and cluck sessions weren't as physically intimate. We would lie on our backs, side by side, holding hands and talking as we always did. The give and take was spirited; we never lacked for that, it was that we just never caressed or stroked each other. Despite her show in public, Ruth's body had taken a beating and she had a lot of physical and mental healing to do.

Intimacy was more for moral support than for physical contact. Although Ruth wasn't usually demonstrative in public, when we were out together she would occasionally pat my arm, or put her hand on my shoulder, or hold my hand. I would pat her cheek, hold her hand, or, when I thought that no one could see us, I would pat her fanny. Touching each other was something that we both needed and craved.

One day we were out doing errands and we stopped at a bar for lunch. We both ordered beer and then Ruth excused herself to go to the lady's room. When she returned, she sat down and noticed that I had taken a sip of my beer. She said, "Why you son of a bitch, you didn't even 'Klunk' with me before you started drinking."

"You are right. My mind was a thousand

miles off. However that is no excuse. I apologize."

We touched glasses, and both of us said, "Klunk, I love you."

Ruth looked at me and said, "I hope that I don't have to retrain you every time I come back from the lady's room."

"I hope so too, but you yourself have missed one or two klunks in the past."

"That's true, but not recently."

That closed the subject but I did make sure that we always klunked from then on.

The first of February marked our fourth wedding anniversary. We went out for supper and I had made arrangements to spend the night at the Marriott, the same hotel where we had stayed over the Fourth of July weekend. We ordered drinks, klunked, and then toasted each other. Ruth said to me, in a forlorn tone, "Honey, I am sorry that this is going to be a dry night for us, I just don't feel in the mood. I feel so badly for you."

I looked at her, stuck my tongue out, and said, "Wife, don't you ever feel sorry for me. A dry night does not bother me, I have other things on my mind at present."

She looked a little dubious. "Well, what is on your mind?"

I smiled, and replied, "I've been thinking

that four years ago today we were wed in Selby Gardens. I was the most fortunate man in the world then, and I still am today. I didn't think it possible that my love could get any sweeter but it has. It's like comparing champagne to gutter water.

"I love you more now than I did even when we first met so long ago. So hush up about this screwing shit. You will get horny again. Trust Me. I married you. I know you.

"If I have any regrets about anything it is that I let you talk me out of getting married in all fifty states of the union. That would have made it impossible to divorce each other and would have gotten us into the Guiness Book of Records. I really wish that we had gotten married in each of the fifty states."

Ruth sat there, a long time, without moving or speaking. Finally, she looked at me and smiled, and said, "Jay, I love you so much. Can we 'klunk' again?" We did.

It was a dry night, but it was an unforgettable night. It was our fourth wedding anniversary. Neither of us knew that our fourth anniversary would be our last anniversary together.

***

The night of February eleventh Ruth and I and

Dottie and Dick went out to dinner to celebrate Ruth's sixty-eighth birthday. Ruth enjoyed the celebration but she always made light of her own birthday. She claimed that, because of her age, she was only celebrating her daughter Tracy's birthday. Both she and Tracy had been born on the same day, February eleventh. Dottie and Dick were always ready to go out with us to eat especially when it was for a celebration. It turned out to be a good evening and two amusing incidents happened that kept me smiling for days.

After our drinks were delivered, Dottie, for the very first time in all the times we had gone out together, noticed that Ruth and I "klunked". The fact that she had not seen us "klunking" before now took Ruth and me by surprise because Dottie is very perceptive and she quickly picks up on anything like that. Especially since we were always open with our ritual toast to each other. Dottie kept asking us if we were sure that we had ever "klunked" in front of her before.

The second incident concerned Ruth's birthday present. I had given her a ring with her birthstone, an amethyst, in the center of the ring. I had presented it to her earlier that day and she had put it on her finger. At dinner, she kept moving her arm, in sweeping gestures, to keep the light reflecting off her amethyst. She looked almost as if she were conducting a symphony orchestra. I had to laugh and I asked her if she ever intended to pick up her silverware. She was really pleased with her ring.

After dinner, we went over to Dick and Dottie's house and continued our celebration. Ruth drank a little wine and I had only one black Russian but we stayed and talked until early the next morning. That day, we did not move very fast or very far. As a matter of fact, it was a good two or three days before Ruth recovered from Tracy's birthday.

From February through May, Ruth began to recover from the side effects of her medical ordeal, and, as she felt better, we began to do more. We enrolled in a beginner's Russian language course at Washtenaw Community College. Neither of us had expected fluency, but we were hoping that by exposure to the language and the Cyrillic Alphabet, we would gain some useful familiarity. We totally underestimated our inability to learn Russian. It wasn't a language you could pick up while doing a crossword puzzle. We became more daunted than enlightened and Ruth began to wonder if picking Russia had been the correct choice.

Of course, by this time it was too late to change our plans. We had already paid for the trip and we had our Russian visas for our passports. There was also a personal complication. On our Costa Rica tour we had made friends with a couple who lived in Ann Arbor. When they found out that we were going to visit Russia, they signed up to take the tour with us. We couldn't back out even if we wanted; we were committed. Despite our second thoughts, the closer we got to our departure date, the more we began to look forward to our trip.

As winter's cold grip ended and the days began to get warmer, the focus of Ruth's life changed. She no longer had daily medical trips for tests or treatments and our calendar started to clear of medical appointments. She did have checkups with both Dr. Curry and Dr. Barnett and she did have lab work done on her blood, but these were becoming more infrequent. All her blood work looked good, so these checkups were scheduled further and further apart.

Ruth felt good and I felt good. We both began to believe that her operation and treatment had been successful. Ruth's hair started to grow back. It began slowly as fuzz, grew to a down, then a stubble, and, finally, into a thick, short hair cap. Ruth watched it grow, checking it often in the mirror and brushing it with her hands.

For over a year Ruth had been like a marble in a maze, rolling down paths that had been laid out by medical science. She had been scourged by chemicals and bombarded by radiation that had scarred and burned her chest. In the process she had lost a breast, she had lost her hair, and she had lost her energy. More important, she felt that she had lost her independence and her femininity. Whatever else she felt she lost, Ruth never lost her hope or her determination. She focused on them throughout her ordeal. Growing hair on her head had a powerful effect upon her both as a person and as a female.

Her physical strength began to return and she could do more without having to stop and rest. In turn, this made her feel better about herself. We began to enjoy all the ordinary tasks most married couples take for granted. All of our activities, no matter how routine, no matter how common, were excursions into normal living. We went about doing our simple duties cloaked in an extraordinary love.

One morning about ten days before our trip, as we were lying in bed, Ruth asked me, "Honey, have you noticed that I have more movement and reach with my left arm? The pain and tenderness are really beginning to go away."

I had seen her trying to flex her arm and exercise it many times, but I had not known that she was making progress. "Ladybug, why don't you try to roll over on your left side? Let's see if we can cuddle."

She moved hesitantly, at first, and then with more confidence as she found that she could maneuver without pain. I turned on my right side, and, for the first time in over eight months we were lying in bed facing each other. I looked into her green eyes and I could see what this ordeal had done to her. It had ravaged her and made her look older, but it had also given her something in return. It had enriched her personality and strengthened her character. Her coping with cancer had made her more attractive, both as a woman and as a person. Thinking this, I said the first thing that came into my head, "Ladybug, wife, I love you."

We spent the next half-hour moving slowly and cautiously. We both wanted to gratify our own feelings and those of our partner, and this was the first time we had tried since Ruth's mastectomy. As we stroked each other we both began to get excited, and Ruth finally said, "Honey, help me get my nightgown off, and be careful, but suck my boob." She was beginning to get over her shame of not having two breasts. I was slow, so as not to hurt Ruth, and I am sure that my leisurely approach aroused her even more. I know it did me. Finally, we were coupled. We both climaxed and then we both lay there, totally spent.

After a while, Ruth said, "Oh honey, I never thought that I would feel horny again. And then I was so afraid that, if I ever did, you would think that I was ugly."

"Ruth, how could I ever think that you are ugly? I know you too well and love you too much to ever think that. As long as I have you I am content; there is nothing else that I want."

We stayed in bed until well after nine o'clock. We were satisfied just to hold each other and talk. When we finally did get up we went for breakfast, drove to the town of Marshall, had dinner at Schuler's restaurant, and came home. It was an ordinary day of living, made special because we wrapped it around each other.

\*\*\*

From that day on, we only looked forward. We had a lot of social events coming up that needed our attention. Our calendar, now almost completely free of medical appointments, started to get cluttered with more satisfying commitments. The biggest of these was our two-week trip to Russia starting at the end of May and we had a lot of preparations to make before we would be ready to go on that trip.

But there were other events that Ruth was just as excited about. We would return from

Russia on Monday, the ninth of June, and Ruth had a fiftieth High School reunion, on the weekend starting Friday, June thirteenth. After the reunion, her brother and his wife were coming to stay for the last weekend in June. Following that, was the Fourth of July weekend, with the fireworks and the family outing at the lake. In addition, after the Fourth of July, there was the possibility that my daughter, Julie, and her husband Michael were going to visit us for a day or two. They would be on their way home from a wedding in Indiana and, if they had time, they were going to make a detour and visit us.

Ruth was eagerly anticipating her high school reunion. She had graduated from University High School, in 1947. University High was a small school supervised by The School of Education of the University of Michigan. Since it was no longer in existence, its memories were all the dearer to those who had gone there. Ruth was looking forward to seeing her former classmates.

There were six or seven women from that class who still lived in this area and they would get together occasionally. When they did meet, they would discuss having a class reunion but nobody ever managed to organize one. Ruth always looked forward to these informal luncheons; she went armed with the latest pictures of her grandchildren. She especially enjoyed the first meeting with her friends after she and I had gotten back together. For that gathering, she went primed with our wedding pictures and stories of our campus days. Surprisingly enough to me, I had met two or three of her friends when Ruth and I were students and I vaguely remembered them.

These ladies would tie up a table for hours talking about the past, the present, and the future. When I said that holding a table prevented the waiter from making money from tips and that didn't seem fair, Ruth agreed with me. But, she said that it wasn't that cut and dried. After lunch, most of the tables were unused until dinner and the ladies always tipped the waiter heavily.

Then, of course, there was the one class member who did not live locally, but who was Ruth's best friend, Mimi. As the plans for the reunion began to be finalized, and information became available, Ruth would call Mimi with the details. She pleaded with Mimi to come to the reunion with Tom and stay at our house. Mimi said that they would definitely try.

After the plans for the reunion started to gel, Ruth decided to go through some of her old photographs and see if she could find any pictures of her classmates. I don't believe Ruth ever threw out a picture in her entire life; she had bags, boxes, bundles, and bales of old pictures. Unfortunately, she had not dated or labeled any of them, so she could not identify most of the people in the pictures. She had to give up because she could not recall who was in each picture. She did stop, not in anger, but in disgust with herself for never having written anyone's name on the picture when it first was taken.

Our private time was even more joyous. Now that Ruth was feeling good physically, and she realized she would not be rejected, she became almost insatiable in her need for intimacy and sex. She claimed she was only fulfilling her wifely duties by responding to my lusty libido. I never said a word. I hoped that I had grown wise enough never to haggle over happiness.

As Ruth's body and soul revived and returned to normalcy, we went about preparing for the trip to Russia. Her major concern was over what clothes to take. Of course, the tour literature gave general guidelines, but the literature also gave warnings about unpredictable weather changes. Ruth would be hesitant to decide what to bring anyhow, but the thought of extremely cold weather made it even harder for her to make up her mind.

After much discussion, we finally decided to approach the problem of what to take from a different angle. We would select the maximum size suitcases allowed and work from there. Necessities, such as toilet kits, medicines, vitamins, and underwear, were put inside the suitcases first. Anything that had to be stored, but still be accessible, such as passports, visas, money, traveler's checks, tickets, and en route medication, was collected and put into our hand carried luggage. Whatever space there was left would be for clothes both stylish and protective. It took a long time to pack our suitcases but at last we were ready.

On May twenty-seventh we left for Russia in high spirits and with great expectations. We flew from Detroit to Boston, and, during our short layover at Logan airport, I tried phoning several friends whom I had not seen since I had left the area in 1992. My timing was bad because not one of them was home and all I could do was leave messages on their answering machines. That was disappointing, as I had been looking forward to catching up on what was going on in their lives. After our layover, we flew from Logan to Frankfurt, changed planes, and then flew on to Moscow.

The Moscow International Airport was dismal, dirty, and depressing. No one from the tour was there to meet us and everyone in the group felt that we had been abandoned. It took us an hour and a half of asking questions in English, to people who spoke only Russian, to find the anthill through which we had to work. Only after we had cleared the massive, hot, confusing, lines of passport controls, customs, and luggage inspection, did anyone meet us and tell us what we should have done. By that time, we were all angry and frustrated. Once we were gathered together we were herded onto busses and taken to our ship, the "Alexey Surkov." Ruth and I felt tired, dirty, and grumpy.

The busses carried us to the Volga River, where our ship was docked. When Ruth and I opened the door to our cabin, our sour mood didn't lighten. The room was so small that sneezing would cause overpressure. The bunks were barely as wide as our shoulders and not even as long as I was tall. They were attached to each wall and there was just enough space between the bunks to get to the head of the bed. It was bigger than our cabin on the Costa Rica boat, but it was still smaller than a gym locker. It was a depressing beginning.

Despite our initial impressions, our tour of Russia turned out to be a total delight. Our three-day stay in Moscow was fascinating. On the first day, as we went to visit Red Square, we quickly discovered that automobile traffic in the downtown area of Moscow, is just as crowded and just as discourteous as the automobile traffic in all of the capitalistic cities.

Red Square was a complete surprise. Whenever I saw it on television, usually on Mayday, there were huge missiles and military troops, marching stolidly in revue before the grim ranks of Communist leaders. It had the appearance of a vast, joyless, panorama. In reality, Red Square is not huge, but it is big, and it is a more cheerful place than it looked on television. The red brick wall of the Kremlin, with its attractive towers, forms one side of the square, and opposite that, the GUM department store takes up the second side of the square. St. Basil's Cathedral and a wide cobble stone road through Red Square form the third side while a historical museum, along with the cobble stone road, forms the fourth side.

There were three facets of Red Square that we were not prepared for. The first was the beauty and the dominance over the rest of the square of St. Basil's Cathedral. The May Day parades would purposely hide the cathedral but its onion shaped colored domes attracted our eyes, and wherever we were on the square, we kept looking back at those dramatic colors. The second was that the Lenin Mausoleum looked so tiny and uninteresting. Even though it was closed, neither Ruth nor I felt any pangs of sorrow that we would not be able to pay our respects. The third was that Red Square was vital and gay, with hordes of tourists and sightseers wandering around. It was a clean, neat, pleasant place and Ruth and I enjoyed it.

The second day we toured Moscow in the morning and Zagorsk, the capital of the Russian Orthodox Church, in the afternoon. Zagorsk was another eye popper with its beautifully colored onion domes and buildings; from a distance it looked almost like DisneyWorld. We went to the Moscow Circus in the evening, and, before going back to our gym locker, we went for a ride on the Moscow subway. We were almost too busy to crawl into our own little bunks but exhaustion finally overwhelmed us.

On the third day, our last day in Moscow, we visited the Kremlin, which also surprised us. It was much larger than we had envisioned. I guess that we didn't take into account that the Kremlin is the center of Russia's huge bureaucratic government. The interior of the Kremlin is much fresher and more attractive than its outside brick walls indicate. The Communists have maintained, and cared for, three or four old, magnificent, churches, and a museum dedicated to the rich trappings of the Tsars. Ruth and I were totally taken aback. The communists themselves were preserving this sybaritic era of Russia's history? We found many startling inconsistencies in facts, deeds, and history, all over this marvelous country. The inconsistencies ranged from the irony of the communists preserving Tsarist trappings to the brutal stupidity of the communist leaders never telling the Russian people how many millions "enemies of the state" Stalin had liquidated. Ruth and I began to be enthralled with this country whose people deserve so much better than they have ever been given by their own past governments.

Before we left Moscow, our tour guide, a handsome woman in her late forties or fifties, gave us a picture of Russian life before "Glasnost". She may have tailored her facts to get bigger tips from her American clients, and for her sake, I certainly hope so. We were surprised to find out just how much of a butcher Joseph Stalin was. The Russians lost at least twenty two million people in the Second World War. That is a staggering figure. However, under the rule of Stalin, and having nothing to do with the Second World War, at least fifteen million more Russians disappeared. That is also a staggering figure. The Russian people would have been better off under the Tsars than they were under the communists. Right now, Russia is so poor that many of her older generation citizens want the communists back in office. From their point of view, I can't blame them. What a long-suffering people the Russian population is.

The next morning, our ship departed from Moscow for our ultimate destination of St. Petersburg. "The Alexey Surkov" traveled about 1,250 kilometers, 770 miles, including a side trip around Lake Onega. Like all the other ships on this waterway, it was an odd ship in that it had a very small draft. It carried 240 passengers and a crew of 130, but it drew less than ten feet of water. That was because much of the waterway was man-made canal, and the ships were designed to avoid hitting shallow bottoms.

We left Moscow on the Moscow River, our first waterway on the trip to St. Petersburg. We went through some canal locks and passed the spire of a "drowned" church. When Stalin ordered the construction of the canal, there were several villages that were below the new water level. Of course the villages disappeared when the canal was completed, as they were flooded out of existence. The "drowned" church is the only visible sign that there were any obstacles in the way of Stalin's progress.

It took us five days to go from Moscow to St. Petersburg. The waterway was made up of rivers, canals, lakes, and reservoirs. We passed through eighteen locks on our journey because Moscow is about 530 feet higher in elevation than St. Petersburg. On board ship, it was sometimes hard to tell where one waterway left off and the next one began. Except that we could make some general observations. The rivers and canals would be narrow and only the canals would have locks to raise and lower the ship. The reservoirs and lakes would be large and, occasionally, the shoreline would be lost in the distance. When we did arrive at St. Petersburg, we anchored in the Neva River.

Along our journey, we made tourist stops at Uglich, Goritsy and Kizhi Island. We spent the day at Petrozavodsk, the capital city of the Karelian Republic and the most northern point of our journey. Petrozavodsk is an industrial city that seemed bleak and grimy, even though it was springtime. Ruth and I wondered what the city would be like in the winter but I think that neither of us really wanted to find out first hand.

That evening, while we were at Petrozavodsk, we went to see the Kantele Folklore Ballet Company and they were absolutely marvelous. They did not dance in the classical ballet style; it was native dancing and native music, fast and wild. It was a pagan ritual compared to classical ballet and it was exhilarating. Our stay was certainly not a waste of time, but Petrozavodsk was not St. Petersburg, and Ruth and I were anxious to move on. Both of us were fascinated by the thought of visiting the Hermitage Museum.

The next morning, we left Petrozavodsk to travel the last of the waterways to St. Petersburg. Ruth and I spent the day relaxing, as there were no more scheduled stops until we arrived at St. Petersburg. We walked the decks, visited with our fellow passengers, lounged in deck chairs, and talked over our trip. I asked Ruth if she were disappointed in our choice of tours. She smiled, patted my arm, and shook her head no. After a moment of silence, she said, "No, Honey, Russia isn't what I expected Russia to be. All my preconceived notions were wrong but I am not at all disappointed. I find myself fascinated with this country. I am enjoying myself."

We steamed on through the evening, and arrived sometime in the early morning of the next day. We were berthed with about ten other ships, all similar in size, shape, and design to our ship. From where were docked, on the outskirts of the city, not much of historic St. Petersburg could be seen. River traffic on the Neva, automobile traffic on the bridges, high rise buildings, apartments, and factories, dominated the landscape. The city looked like any other large city that had a population of five million.

Once we were bussed downtown that all changed. The charm and beauty of St. Petersburg enveloped and surrounded us immediately; it was like stepping into a rose garden in full bloom. Our first day in Petersburg was spent touring the city. The weather was a gorgeous warm day full of sunshine and high spirits. In fact, the only bad weather we had on the entire trip was an afternoon of rain in Petrozavodsk. We toured all over downtown St. Petersburg as we visited Tsarist palaces, public buildings and museums. We were driven past monuments to Russian intellectuals and Peter the Great, churches, cathedrals, and the cruiser "Aurora", where the Russian revolution had begun. We crossed over countless bridges that spanned the canal system that weaves through St. Petersburg.

Ruth and I were intoxicated by the city. Everything was scrupulously clean. The churches and cathedrals were riots of color. The buildings were massive, old, and handsome. Everything was beautiful on the outside and glittering on the inside. The gilded opulence absolutely astounded us.

By late afternoon, we were toured out and sated by the wonders we had seen. We were on the bus headed back to our ship, in preparation for a visit to the ballet that evening. As we relaxed, and chatted, it became obvious that Ruth and I had been having similar thoughts as we were sightseeing. What we had seen, so far, had been breathtaking.

However, we both wondered about the run down and seedy parts of St. Petersburg. Surely, like every large metropolis, there must be uninviting sections to this city. Had all the damage from the Second World War been repaired, or just here where the visitors came? After all, the Germans had laid siege to this city, then called Leningrad, for almost 900 days. The pain and suffering inflicted on the inhabitants of Leningrad had been unbearable. One third of the city had been destroyed by bombardment during the siege. Over one million of the inhabitants had perished from either starvation or being frozen to death. We were in awe of the St. Petersburg we did see, but we wondered about the St. Petersburg we did not see.

The next day, Friday, we were scheduled to visit the Hermitage Museum in the morning and Peter the Great's Summer Palace in the afternoon. The weather was warm and sunny, a bright, happy day. We were bussed to Palace Square, a huge, open area, surrounded by massive, three and four storied buildings, one of which was the Hermitage. There, our tour group waited, along with twenty or thirty other large tour groups, for admittance into the museum. The Hermitage had been one of the major attractions that had tempted us to make this trip.

While we were waiting, everyone in the crowd was subjected to hawkers, peddlers, mendicants, and beggars. A very small gypsy boy, about four or five years old, would kneel in front of a tourist, put his hands together on his chest, just below his chin, and pray for money. It was shocking and pitiful, and, if the tourist tried to ignore him, he would rock back and forth and plead even louder. Eventually, the victim would be so embarrassed that he, or she, would give the kneeling, wailing child some money just to get rid of him.

When the gypsy boy started working our group, he knelt in front of the wife of a retired U of M professor. Her husband had just given her a 500-ruble note, worth about ten cents in our currency, to spend when she went to the lady's room. It is customary, and necessary, in Russia to tip the attendant in the public bathrooms in order to get a few sheets of toilet paper. In her haste to get rid of the gypsy boy, the woman mistakenly grabbed the 500-ruble note, and gave it to him. While he knelt, he looked at it, crumpled it up, and just threw it down on the pavement. His brother, older by one or two years, ran over, picked it up, spoke harshly in a language we did not understand to the younger boy, and pocketed the 500 rubles. It must be that even the gypsies believe that they are entitled to a minimum wage.

After being in the square for an hour, we entered the Hermitage, and we were told that picture taking inside the museum would be forbidden to the general public. However, if any individual really wanted to take pictures, he could, for a price, purchase a camera permit. Once you purchased a permit, you were allowed to take pictures of anything and everything. I wanted the option of being able to photograph the French Impressionist paintings, so I was glad to purchase one of their camera permits. Although I did take some pictures inside the Hermitage, I did not take any pictures of paintings. I started to become concerned as to whether or not all the flashes and strobes could damage those beautiful and irreplaceable works of art. Not knowing, I stopped taking pictures just to be sure.

The Hermitage exceeded our expectations. We were entranced, almost in a daze. The exhibitions were stunning. Room after room after room of furniture, paintings, and furnishings were on display. It was hard to believe that so many gorgeous masterpieces could be assembled in one location. We could easily have spent a week looking at everything in the museum, but we didn't have that kind of time.

The French Impressionist paintings were as beautiful as we had hoped, and anticipated, that they would be. We wanted to take our time and look at each painter and each of his paintings. That is what we had done when we went to see the Monet exhibit at the Chicago Museum. In Chicago, we went at our own pace, however, in St. Petersburg, we were not that fortunate. Our tour guide was like a cowboy on a cattle drive, she herded, harassed, and hurried us. She was as gentle as possible but it was her job to keep us dogies moving. So she kept busy, rounding us up in a quiet, polite, firm way. She did a good job of cajoling and pushing us along.

With all the people that were inside the building, and the warm weather outside, the museum got hot. The building did not seem to have any air conditioning or at least none that could handle that size a crowd under such warm weather conditions. I kept wondering what the temperature and humidity was going to do to those precious paintings. Anything that is beautiful in this world deserves to be protected.

After lunch at a downtown restaurant, we went, by bus, just outside of St. Petersburg, to Peter the Great's Summer Palace, on the Gulf of Finland. It was similar to the other palaces that we had seen in St. Petersburg; huge, opulent, edifices filled with objets d'art. It was a splendid monument to the unbridled life style of the Tsars.

What made it absolutely fascinating for me was the fact that it was a complete and total reproduction. The original Summer Palace had been entirely destroyed by the Nazis in World War II. They had never entered Leningrad, but they had overrun the Summer Palace. When they were forced to retreat, they maliciously burnt the Palace down. After the war ended the communists had carefully reproduced everything that we saw, the buildings, the inlaid floors, and the furnishings.

It had been a painful, thorough, slow and costly rebuilding process. The ashes had been sifted to identify the types of wood that had been used in building the original Summer Palace. Old plans, old pictures, and archives were studied to ensure the accuracy of the new Summer Palace. The Russian government spared no expense in eradicating the wanton desecration of one of their national treasures. What they accomplished is truly a marvel.

When we finished our tour of the Summer Palace, we strolled back to our bus, which was parked outside the huge gardens that surround the palace. As we neared the parking area, we passed through a small tent city of merchants selling tourist trash. Souvenirs, wristwatches, cold drinks, postcards, and T-shirts were on sale. We had passed through this group of entrepreneurs on our way in, but we had been in a hurry and had paid scant attention to what was being offered for sale. Now that we were on our way out, we spent some time examining their wares. The hottest selling item was the wooden, lacquered dolls that nested inside each other. These matrushka dolls, however, weren't painted with the traditional Russian themes. Instead, they portrayed the Chicago Bulls basketball team. The largest doll was of Michael Jordan the smaller dolls nesting inside the Jordan doll were of Scotty Pippin, Dennis Rodman, and the rest of the team. Ruth and I laughed at the idea that people would travel all the way over to Russia to buy souvenirs of the Chicago Bulls. American capitalism had come to communist Russia.

That evening, Ruth and I walked on the deck of our ship just as the sun was setting. It was warm and clear and we stood with our elbows on the rail. Ruth slipped her hand into mine, and said, "Jay, I can't believe all the beauty we have seen on this trip. I see it, I enjoy it, and I wonder why there has to be so much hate and ugliness in this world. I think I am happier and more content right now than I was even on our Alaskan trip." She patted my hand and kissed me on the cheek. For once, I had no answer. I did not need one. I was content. We stood there, side by side, savoring the day, savoring the memories, and savoring one another. Ruth sighed, and added, "I just wish that our bunks didn't make this a no screwing ship. C'mon, let's go get a beer."

The following morning, Saturday, we were on our own. There was a canal tour of St. Petersburg at 2:00PM that we had signed up to take, but we had decided against taking an optional tour of another palace in the morning. The Summer Palace had left us emotionally and aesthetically drained. For the first time on our trip, our boat was docked and we had a leisurely morning in which to relax and enjoy ourselves without having anywhere to go.

After talking it over at breakfast, and asking our guides, we decided to take one of our tour busses to downtown St. Petersburg, find a place to eat, and eventually wander over to where the canal tour departed. At first, Ruth was hesitant and wanted to wait for the tour bus that would bring us right to where the canal tour started. Her concern was not that we couldn't speak Russian, it was that we might get lost and miss going on the canal ride.

At first, I wasn't so sure myself. Neither of the two maps that I looked at showed the bridge, where the boat started the tour, at the same place. I pointed out the discrepancy to the purser and he finally admitted that, while one of the maps had to be wrong, he wasn't sure which

map it was. He checked, and eventually pro-
duced a third map that was more detailed than
the other two and showed the exact location of
the bridge. I assured Ruth that I would get us to
the bridge in time to board the boat. That was all
she needed, as she was anxious to walk around
and get the flavor of St. Petersburg.

The bus dropped us off in front of the Hotel Astoria. Since this was the final day of our
trip, and since we were scheduled to spend the
next night at this hotel, we were curious about
it. Our tour information said that it was a four
star hotel and we wanted to see what a four star
hotel looked like, so we decided to go in and look
around.

The only way you could enter the lobby
was by passing through a metal detecting machine, similar to those used in airports. When
Ruth saw the machine, she pulled me to a stop.
She said, "We are going to set that machine off.
Why would they have you pass through a metal
detector to enter a four star hotel?"

I certainly didn't know. "Maybe we should
stay at a three star hotel instead," was all that
I could answer. We stood in the same spot, and
watched what was going on for a few minutes.
Everyone who went through the machine triggered the alarm. It rang constantly.

Finally, I said, "Maybe this is part of the

local custom. If you don't set the alarm off, you get arrested. Let's go through anyhow, and see what happens on the other side."

Of course we set it off and nobody seemed to care. We found that the lobby was handsome, modern, and clean. Absolutely no one paid the slightest attention to the alarm, which was going off continuously. We were told later that the security people were only looking for known Russian Mafia members. Ruth and I decided that it didn't make any difference to us whether the alarm got triggered or not, as long we didn't get involved.

We left the Astoria and started to walk towards the bridge where our canal tour would begin. The temperature was over eighty degrees, and after a few minutes, we were both hot. We came across a small park near the magnificent Church of the Blood, so we went in to sit on a bench for a few minutes as we has plenty of time to get to our destination.

As we were sitting and chatting a young man walked by us, stopped, and returned to stand in front of us. He said, "I apologize for interrupting you, but aren't you Americans?" Ruth smiled at him and replied, "Yes, my husband and I are Americans. Are you?"

"Yes, I am and I am so glad to meet Americans. My name is Jim Brant and I have been on a missionary tour for two years in Eastern Russia in a town called Yamsk. It is a bleak place, but it's full of really nice people.

"Anyhow, I am nearing the end of my mission. My mother and father are flying into St. Petersburg from Utah. They will be here tonight and that is why I am hoping that you can help me. Where can I find out what operas and concerts, and things like that are being done in St. Petersburg in the next few days?"

We both smiled; talk about the blind leading the lame. Ruth answered his question, "We would be glad to try to help you, but you have asked two people who have been in St. Petersburg for just two and a half days. Our first night here, we went to see the Nutcracker ballet, so I know that the Ballet Company is performing, but I do not know their schedule. Why don't you go to one of the large hotels, like the Astoria, and speak to the concierge? I am sure that a concierge can tell you all the events that are going on. That is the only suggestion that I can make."

He beamed. "Thank you, thank you," he said. "That is an excellent suggestion."
He chatted with us for about twenty minutes before he left. He was a young, enthusiastic, person who was homesick and looking forward to being reunited with his mother and father. We

enjoyed our conversation with him. After he left, we got up from the bench and continued on our journey.

About two blocks away from the bridge we were heading to, we stopped at a courtyard that had a heavy iron fence across the front of it. The gate was swung wide open and there was an advertisement for a restaurant inside the gate, so we entered the courtyard. There were twelve to fifteen tables with big umbrellas to block out the sun and the tables were almost completely filled. It didn't really matter, as they only served drinks in the courtyard, the restaurant itself was on the second floor of a building that faced the courtyard. We made our way up a wide staircase and entered the restaurant, which was partitioned into small rooms. There were only a few customers.

The waitress handed us menus and started to speak to us in Russian. Ruth looked at me and rolled her eyes upward, and I had to agree with her unspoken comment. We might be in trouble. The waitress tried to be helpful, but she flipped through the menu so fast and spoke so rapidly, that neither of us could get the gist of what she meant. Finally, the waitress walked away. Ruth and I studied the menus, which were written in Russian, and then we looked at each other.

A woman walked over to our table. "Hello," she said. "Olga told me that she is having difficulty with you."

"And we with her," I replied. "We do not speak Russian and she does not speak English. The language barrier makes it hard to communicate. We would like to order a light lunch and some cold beer. We would certainly appreciate any help you could give us."

"That is no problem. Let me recommend a few items for you and see if you agree."

Thus began an excellent lunch and a fascinating conversation. The woman, whose name neither Ruth nor I could remember later, was an American who had settled in St. Petersburg. She had opened the first Pizza Hut in St. Petersburg and had recently sold it to buy this restaurant. The restaurant itself was located in an apartment that had belonged to a long time conductor of the St. Petersburg Symphony Orchestra.

We learned all of this during our delightful meal of borscht, toss salad, roast pork sandwich and Russian beer. The owner came over to talk to us in between her chores. We had stumbled into a pleasant interlude.

When we left the restaurant we walked over to the bridge where the canal tour was going to depart. We arrived about twenty minutes before the boat left and watched as the rest of our group straggled in. The tour of the "Venice of the North" was another trip into a landscape of loveliness. We saw all of the same landmarks that we had seen before, but our perspective was entirely different. The buildings, the churches, the castles, the bridges we went under, all were beautiful as seen from our canal boat. It was memorable, and yet, everyone on board was glad when the tour finished.

The problem was the heat. The sun beat down on our boat and soon, the temperature inside the glass-covered cabin became almost unbearable. It must have been over 100 degrees where we were seated. The entire group on board was hot, tired, and wet with sweat by the time the boat returned to the bridge. The first thing that Ruth and I did when we went onboard the "Alexey Surkov" was to down a cold Russian beer.

We sat around telling our friends about our adventures of the day. How we had set off the metal detector in the Astoria, how we had helped a young missionary find his way in St. Petersburg, and how we had had such an interesting luncheon experience. We attracted quite an audience before we finished. I gather most everyone considered Ruth and me an amusing, if not offbeat, senior couple.

That evening, we had a farewell cocktail party for everyone in our University of Michigan travel group. The party marked the end of the tour. The next day, Sunday, June eight, most of the group went to the airport and departed for their various destinations. For some reason, the people flying to Detroit were held over one night and would leave early Monday morning, instead of sometime Sunday.

We were transported to the Astoria on Sunday, put up for the night, and scheduled to be at the airport for a 5:30AM flight on Monday. Since the advertised rate for our room was $260 a night, we were curious to see if we could find any differences between a four star hotel and the no star motels where we had always stayed before. We certainly did find differences.

The room was clean, airy, and elegant. We examined it thoroughly, and could find no fault. It was lavishly supplied with fresh flowers, bottles of oils, soaps, lotions, and, for each of us to wear after our showers, heavy terry cloth bathrobes.

We had an elegant early supper in the hotel dining room as we had a 4:30 AM wake up call. We dined with a few of the other tour couples, said goodbye to those not traveling home with us, and retired to our room.

After we had each cleaned up, Ruth and I lounged around wearing our hotel bathrobes and sipping wine. Ruth asked me, "Do you like your robe, Honey. Do you want to buy one and take it home?"

I replied, "I like this robe, Ladybug. But not enough that I would want to either buy it or steal it. How about you? Are you interested in buying one?"

"No, Honey, I don't want to take one home either. They are fun to wear, but they are too heavy for me.

"Listen, I will tell you one thing that I finally found to be disappointed about. For the price of this room, I was hoping that the bath arrangement would allow both of us to shower together. We haven't done that since one of our trips to Niagara Falls. But with that high-walled tub, and that hand-held shower wand, it wouldn't be much fun soaping each other.

"Still, I can't get over how nice this room is. Do you think it was like this during the Communist era?"

"I would guess so, Ruth. There were always visitors from other nations coming into Leningrad, or St. Petersburg, or whatever they called this town. And they had to stay somewhere. Keeping them in places like this would make it easy for the Communists to keep track of visitors and spy on them."

Ruth repeated my last words. "Spy on them?"

"Sure, my hunch is that they would bug these rooms to watch their guests and hear them. I am sure that, if we could have, we would have done the same thing to suspicious foreigners when they came to our country."

"You mean that right now, in this room, there could be cameras that are letting people watch and listen to us?"

"Possibly there could be, but probably not. If we are being spied on, they might have seen both of us while we were taking our showers."

Ruth sniffed, "Well, I don't like that idea at all." We changed the subject to talk about our early departure in the morning, and then went to bed.

We lay there snuggling. I was rubbing her just below the small of her back, when Ruth asked, "Honey, do you think this room is bugged?"

"I don't really think so, Ladybug, but it could be. And that is too bad because all those nights aboard the boat have made me horny."

Ruth sighed, "I think it is a terrible country where two married people don't have the privacy to do whatever they want. Even in Costa Rica we managed to do it. I will be glad to get back to our own bedroom. I have decided that communism was a very evil form of government."

We lay there for a while and Ruth began

to nibble gently on my neck. I began to rub her backside. "Of course," Ruth began, "they would not see anything that they haven't seen before. I hope that they aren't watching, but shame on them if they are. Why should we stop our normal activities because they are so filthy minded?"

We kept snuggling and rubbing; we were both getting excited. Ruth said, "To hell with them. If they want to watch two American geezers screwing, let's show them what we can do. It's almost our patriotic duty, and I want to, so lets have at it."

We did our best.

The next morning, at 5:30 AM, we left our hotel. We thought that we were on our way home; we were not. We were heading straight toward the valley of the shadow of death. Ruth had only thirty-five days more to live.

## WINTER

Our return trip was an absolute horror show. We encountered unexpected delays on every leg of the return trip. We left Moscow at 5:30 AM on Sunday, June eighth and didn't get back to Detroit Metropolitan Airport until 4:00 PM on Monday. When the seven-hour time difference between Moscow and Detroit is subtracted out, Ruth and I were traveling for almost thirty hours. Much of the time was spent in airports waiting between flights. During the long trek, we both got little sleep and we ate unappetizing snacks. When we finally did reach our house, we were tired, dirty and grateful to be home.

Ruth's high school reunion was scheduled to start on Friday. We had known before we left that we would have only three days between our arrival home and the start of her reunion. However, there was no alternative if we were going to go to Russia, and we could never have imagined the exhausting return trip. We had planned to spend those three days relaxing and recovering, and of course, nothing went according to our plans.

Our friends called wanting to know about our trip and how Ruth was doing; my daughters called wanting to know about our trip and how Ruth was doing; Ruth's daughters came over wanting to know about our trip and how Ruth was doing. We spent hours continuously repeating details and answering the same questions over and over. Meanwhile, our chores, errands, and preparations for the reunion kept getting delayed.

None of these distractions would have been of any importance at all except that Ruth told me she felt a little tired. The long trip home had taken its toll on her and she also thought that she might have picked up a bug. She said that she had an appointment scheduled with Dr. Curry early on Friday morning, and when she saw the doctor, she would tell her about feeling tired. I was a little concerned but I wasn't worried. Ruth had done well during our trip and I thought that she had what I had, a little jet lag.

Friday turned out to be a busy day. In the morning, we both went to Dr. Curry's office. She gave Ruth a thorough examination and ordered some blood work done. After her exam, we drove over to Ann Arbor to pick up a minivan we had rented for the reunion weekend. Our station wagon was beginning to show its age, and Ruth and I had been talking about buying a minivan for months. We decided to rent one over a weekend, and compare it to a station wagon. We chose this weekend because Mimi and Tom were coming from California and staying at our house. Our minivan would be our transportation and it would also give us a chance to make a thorough comparison.

At the last moment, just before leaving California, Mimi and Tom decided to stay at a hotel in Ann Arbor. The decision was in deference to our schedule and Ruth's illness. Ruth was disappointed, but she realized that their plan was more practical than our idea had been. Wherever they stayed, the four of us would still drive together to the reunion events in our rented minivan.

After we picked it up, I drove home and Ruth rested a little. The first event of the weekend was a buffet dinner and cocktail party at Joan Innes's house in Ann Arbor. Joan and Ruth had been friends since childhood and Joan had been in one or two of my classes when we were both going to college.

Mid afternoon on Friday, we got ready and went over to the hotel to see Mimi and Tom. We had not seen them since our wedding and we had a lot of talking, and catching up, to do. It was a beautiful June day, warm, sunny, and fragrant with the promise of summer. We found a little bar near the university campus, and as we sat at a small table, the two ladies babbled sweetly and innocently like water running over rocks. Fifty years of friendship can neither be dammed nor denied. Tom and I looked at each other, shrugged our shoulders, and held our own conversation, as there was no room for us to intrude on theirs. We talked until it was time to get ready for the cocktail party. The four of us walked back to the hotel, freshened up in Mimi and Tom's hotel room, and then drove over to the Innes household.

The cocktail party was a happy, exciting event. Large name tags helped everyone recall the names of their classmates without staring too much. University High had been a small school; there were only about fifty or sixty students in Ruth's senior class. And even though fifty years had passed, the names and the memories were quickly recalled and they brought nostalgia and joy to the class of 1947. Meetings between classmates, separated for so long, sparked stories and gales of laughter. These, in turn, triggered other stories, other memories, and more laughter. The little mysteries and misunderstandings of fifty years were cleared up and dissolved in the camaraderie that age brings to survivors.

Even as a spousal outsider, I had a hell of a good time. They were an interesting group of people. There were a lot of professors, lawyers, doctors, authors, and teachers among them.

They were genuinely interested in each other's fortunes. Even though I didn't share in their inside jokes, they made me feel welcome and I enjoyed talking with them.

When the party was over, we dropped Mimi and Tom off at their hotel and we went home. As we were driving, I asked Ruth how she was doing. She laughed and said that she had a marvelous time seeing her old classmates, but that she felt a little tired.

Saturday morning we both woke up slowly, and, as we cooed and clucked, Ruth said, "Honey, I didn't sleep too well. I kept waking up with night sweats."

That struck me as odd. She should have been over all her travel aches and pains by this time. I asked, "Ladybug, how do you feel right now?"

She snuggled closer to me and answered, "Right now, I feel fine but I think that I want to take it kind of easy today. I'm really looking forward to our class dinner this evening. I hope it will be as much fun as the cocktail party."

We did take it easy for the rest of the day. I ran errands and Ruth did what she needed to do over the phone. The hotel that was catering the dinner was the same Marriott where we had spent both the Fourth of July and our anniversary celebration. When Mimi and Tom realized where the dinner was, Mimi called to tell us not to come to Ann Arbor just to pick them up and then drive right back to Ypsilanti. They had rented a car to visit their friends and family and they would use it to meet us at the Marriott. Ruth agreed and used this extra time to rest a little more. We were ready to go early so we drove over to the hotel to get a drink and visit with whomever showed up.

The dinner wasn't nearly as much fun as the cocktail party. We were seated in a huge banquet room and the room seated many more people than were attending our banquet. That would not have made much difference except that, in addition to being oversized, the room was dimly lit and the food was cold and not very appetizing. Disappointment cast a pall over the group making the dinner a very quiet affair.

Worse than that, nothing had been scheduled after the meal. There were no rooms reserved, and no one had made any plans for getting together when we finished eating. As a result, we came into the banquet room, we ate quickly and soberly, and, for a while, we milled around in the hall outside the banquet room. People began to leave simply because there was nothing else to do. Ruth and I chatted with individual couples, but soon there was no one left with whom to talk; they had straggled out of the hotel in small groups. Compared with the exuberant cocktail party Friday night, Saturday's dinner was a dismal failure. Disappointed, we were home and in bed by midnight.

Sunday morning Ruth was still tired and she had had more night sweats. I became worried, something was not right. Ruth knew it and I knew it; but since she didn't say anything more, I didn't ask any more questions.

Sunday turned out to be another beautiful, sunny day. We picked up Mimi and Tom and drove out to Independence Lake, where the picnic was being held. It was a pretty location and every one was in a good mood. The damp spirit of the last evening evaporated in the bright sunshine and the pleasant surroundings. Ruth had as good a time at the picnic as she had at the cocktail party. She mingled, rehashed the past, laughed, told stories, and listened to the stories of her classmates. She slaked her fifty-year memory thirst and enjoyed herself doing it.

Late in the afternoon, we drove Mimi and Tom back to their hotel in Ann Arbor. We went up to their room to talk and make plans because Mimi and Tom would be departing for California in the morning and we wanted to try to get together again as soon as possible. We promised to meet sometime in the coming year, and they invited us to use their cottage in Carmel anytime. We had stayed in that cottage one weekend after I had finally sold the house in California. We were thrilled by their offer because we had had such a good time in Carmel. We embraced, kissed, and said our goodbyes. For some odd reason I thought, "This is Sunday, June fifteenth and today is Father's Day."

After we got home, Ruth told me that she was tired. I knew part of that was a let down after seeing all of her classmates. But I also knew that something was wrong. We lolled around the house the rest of the day and went to bed early that evening.

Monday morning as we cooed and clucked, Ruth told me that she felt good. She had slept soundly and had had no night sweats. Now she said, she had to plan for Joan and Edward's visit, the Fourth of July picnic, and the visit from Julie and her family. I was relieved to hear her being so chatty.

I returned the rented minivan to Ann Arbor early in the morning. By the time I returned it was after 9:00A.M. Ruth and I were sitting together, working on a shopping list, when the phone rang. Ruth answered it, and I watched her as she listened. She finally said, "O.K., call me back when you have the time of the examination."

She hung up, looked at me, and said, "Oh,

poop."

I asked her, "What was that all about?"

"That was Dr. Curry's office. They called to tell me that some of my blood tests are not normal. They want to do a CAT scan, so they're going to set up an appointment and call me right back."

Ruth looked at me and I looked at her. With that simple statement we both realized that neither her chemotherapy treatments nor her radiation treatments had been successful. Ruth still had cancer.

She sat quietly for a few minutes, and then said abruptly, "Shit, I have to go to the bathroom." She stood up and walked out of the room.

I was stunned. I didn't know what to do, I didn't know what to say, I didn't know what to think. I just sat there. Almost half an hour went by before I realized that Ruth was still in the bathroom. I walked by the closed door three or four times before I asked, "Ruth? Are you coming out soon?"

She replied, "I'll be out in a few minutes. Go sit down and quit pacing."

I went back to the dinette table and sat. Ruth came out of the bathroom a short time later. As she came near me I took hold of her hand and squeezed it. I said to her, "I love you Ruth.

Are you all right?"

Ruth reacted angrily. She said, "Well what do you think? I finally get to Easy Street and now I won't be able to enjoy it." She stopped and looked at me. "No, that is wrong. We have had such a good time. Oh, Honey, I feel so sorry for you. You got the shitty end of the stick."

I thought, "How can she say that? Why should she say that?" I took a deep breath. I said, "Ladybug, that is not true. I did not get the shitty end of the stick. I have no complaints."

Rising from my chair, I stood beside Ruth and she turned to meet me. We held each other loosely and swayed back and forth, almost as if we were dancing. Ruth put her head on my shoulder.

"I love you, wife."

"And I love you, Jay Carp. But you listen to me we are going to have some new ground rules around here. Do you hear me?"

"Yes, I hear you, Ruth. What are they?"

She took her head off my shoulder, stood up straight, and held my hands in hers. She looked at me and said, "You are not to cry. Honey, I am going to need all the strength I have. You have got to help me by being strong for me and with me. I need that Honey. I don't know if I can be brave without you. Please help me."

I didn't trust myself to speak. I was choked

up. I just nodded, yes. Ruth smiled, "Thank you. Next, we tell the kids, both yours and mine, as little as possible. We don't know anything for certain and we will only deal with facts. We will parcel out information to them and everyone else only when we have those facts."

Again I nodded.

"And last, I guess I want to live as normally as possible. My brother and Joan are coming, we have our Fourth of July picnic, and Julie will be arriving. I don't want to cancel anything. They are all important to me. I need to enjoy whatever I can."

I was finally able to ask, "Anything else, Ladybug?"

Ruth said, "No." She thought a second, smiled a little, and then added, "Not right now. But, if I do think of anything else, I'll let you know."

Trying to answer her back in kind, I replied, " I have absolutely no doubt that you will."

Later that day, Dr. Curry's office called back and gave Ruth an appointment for her CAT scan. It was scheduled the day before her brother arrived, eleven days from now, the twenty-seventh of June.

That evening, lying in bed, neither of us could sleep, and neither of us felt like talking. We just held hands, each of us churning and chewing on our own sour, bitter thoughts. Finally, as Ruth fell asleep, she said, in a tiny voice, "Oh Honey, don't let anything bad happen to me."

I lay there without moving; I was wracked with pain, sorrow and fury. I could not help my beloved wife. We were both subjects of fate and neither of us controlled what was going to happen. We were helpless and hopeless.

Ruth had asked me not to cry and I wanted to do what she needed me to do. I kept biting the inside of my mouth until it began to bleed a little. I was afraid of rousing Ruth if I tried to get out of bed, so I lay still. I wanted to cry, I wanted to scream, I wanted so desperately to help Ruth, yet there was nothing I could do.

I couldn't reconcile anything. Why was this happening? Why wasn't God more careful with his treasures? If God had a complaint about me, and He had many reasons to be unhappy, why not punish me directly? Why hurt someone who was so much better than I? Ruth had never knowingly harmed anyone, and she had helped so many. There are so many mean, nasty, people in this world, why take away someone who is loved and needed? The time we had spent together was not enough; we both wanted more. We both deserved more.

I felt desolate. There is no God. Life is just a random series of incidents. It is up to each individual person to try to bring order out of chaos and find whatever solace and happiness he or she can.

Ruth's plea echoed in my mind, over and over, again and again. Throughout that long, unhappy night I heard that tiny voice repeating, "Oh Honey, don't let anything bad happen to me."

I was going to fail Ruth because I was powerless to help. I was squeezed by pain and suffering; pressed into the mattress like a ship on the floor of the ocean. Finally, the birds began to sing and I fell asleep.

\*\*\*

I awoke with a start. At first I was disoriented. Ruth's side of the bed was empty and I got frightened. I didn't know where she was or what she was doing. I jumped up, put on my bathrobe, and hurried out of the bedroom. Ruth was sitting at the dinette table with a writing pad, a pen, and a cup of coffee, in front of her.

She said, "Well Lazy Head, you finally woke up. I was beginning to wonder about you."

Seeing her sitting at her usual location, doing her ordinary tasks, calmed my fears. I patted her on the shoulder and kissed her on the top of her head.

"Grab yourself a cup of coffee and come sit down. I need your help planning for the Ormondroyds, the picnic, and the Harlows."

After pouring my coffee, I sat down opposite her. She looked at me closely, for a second, and then she asked, "Honey, what is wrong with your face? Your mouth looks a little swollen."

I had no intention of telling Ruth about the night I had gone through, instead I said, "I think I must have had a bad dream and I bit my lip a little. I don't remember much about the dream, but I do remember biting my lip."

"Well, I hope it isn't as tender as it looks. Listen, help me a little and then I'll get breakfast for both of us. I am trying to figure out what to bring to the lake and what to serve for Ed and Joan and Julie and Michael."

I was lost. I had no idea of what to suggest nor was I really interested. I couldn't get that phone call from the doctor out of my mind. I sipped my coffee and finally began, "Are you sure that you want to go through with all of this? I could call Julie and Michael and ask them not to visit."

Ruth shook her head and said, "No Honey that is exactly what is not going to happen. You and I both know what is going on, and I am not going to stop doing what I want to do. These are probably my last visits and my last picnic. I want to have them and I will have them. I maybe forced to slow down, but I am not going to stop."

"How about having Christie and Tracy come over and help you clean up the house and get ready?"

"Jay, in all the years that I have lived in this house, I have never had anyone do my cleaning for me. This is my home and I will take care of it. I will not have my daughters, or anyone else, do my work for me. I will hold on as long as I possibly can."

Her pride and courage stopped me from making any other suggestions. "Ladybug, everything will be done exactly as you say. So, let's get on to the next point. What do you want from me?"

Ruth sat quietly for a while. She looked at me with those beautiful green eyes of hers, and then, in a low voice, she said, "You will have the most important job of all. I want you to be near me, I want your support, I want your love. I need you now like I have never needed anyone before."

How to reply? How do you reassure the person who means everything to you? I took a deep breath. "Ruth, Honey, these things are already yours. I gave them to you when I told you that I loved you.

"I will be here because I adore you. I am absolutely crazy about you."

"You may be crazy, Honey, but it sure is in a nice way. I am so glad that you came back to me."

We went on to discuss the details of what she wanted to do for our families and for the picnic. I was able to convince her to cut down on some of her plans but it wasn't easy. Ruth wanted to keep her activities as close to normal as possible and I wanted her to conserve her strength as much as possible. We would talk, I would recommend, she would decide. Once she decided, I stopped discussing. I wanted to help her, not harass her.

The intervening days that we had before her CAT scan, from the sixteenth until the twenty-seventh were like living in the eye of a hurricane. We knew that we were surrounded by a terrible turbulence, but we were becalmed. We were never closer. It was as if our minds were tuned to the same wavelength. I knew what her thoughts were, and she knew mine. We couldn't, and didn't, hide our fears, our concerns, or our love. And, despite what we knew the future would bring, our life was as sweet as the center of a watermelon.

Ruth wasn't in any pain. She had night sweats and stomach discomfort. Her only external symptoms were that her belly began to swell and her appetite started to decline.

I didn't ask her how she was feeling but I watched her closely and tried to help her whenever she would let me. She kept up her normal duties cleaning, cooking, running errands and visiting with her daughters. She and I both knew that it was a strain for her but she would have it no other way. Ruth just would not quit.

We both needed to keep active just to carry on. Ruth would walk by where I was sitting and pat my shoulder. Then she would look at me and smile. I knew that she was worried and that touching me made her feel better. I did not miss any chance to caress her cheek or kiss her hair. These contacts were not preludes to anything; they were simple gestures of love and respect and conveyed our feelings for each other.

Our nights were our best times. We went to bed early, because Ruth would be tired, and we would coo and cluck. We talked and laughed and held each other. Neither of us mentioned Ruth's CAT scan but we both knew it was coming. We turned to each other and merged our feelings. I guess we were hoping that our love would ward off evil and keep us together. We hid inside of our love until the day of her appointment.

Friday, the twenty-seventh of June, at 1:10 in the afternoon, we went to the hospital for the

CAT scan. It was a hot, sunny day, and the heat took its toll on Ruth. Before the procedure began, she had to drink a large amount of medicine. For once she complained about both the taste of what she had to swallow and what she had to go through. It seemed to take a long time before the procedure was completed. When she came out of the room she was tired and quiet. On the way home she said, "Jay, you should never have returned to Ann Arbor. You got a bad deal."

I reached over and patted her knee but I didn't answer her. She hardly spoke a word all evening.

Joan and Edward arrived Saturday. They came to Ann Arbor every year to visit Ruth and see their friends. Edward had gone to University High also but he had graduated two years before Ruth.

For Saturday's meal, we stayed home and I made spaghetti. Sunday, I drove Joan and Edward to Murray Lake to see Christie and Tracy and all of the grandchildren. Ruth stayed home to rest. Robin was not there as she had moved to Atlanta. She would not be back in Ypsilanti either for this weekend or for the Fourth of July picnic.

That evening, Ruth, Edward, Joan and I spent time chatting and reminiscing about Mrs. O, Professor O, and Ruth and Edward's childhood memories. Ruth was pleased that she and her brother were closer now than they had ever been before.

Joan planted the rest of the remaining flats of flowers that Ruth had bought earlier in the month and had never put into the ground. Ruth was gratified and touched when she saw the planting Joan had done. I think Ruth used the visit to purge herself of some of the bad feelings she had towards her childhood.

I spent most of my time watching Ruth because I was sure that she was not feeling well. The CAT scan had upset her both mentally and physically, and I thought she was having some physical discomfort. According to her rules, I could watch her but I couldn't ask questions. Even our coo and cluck sessions were subdued. It wasn't a good weekend.

Early Monday morning, Joan and Edward started back to New York. Just before 10:00AM, Ruth got a call from Dr. Curry's office. Dr. Curry wanted to talk to us as soon as possible. We made an appointment for late that afternoon.

When we arrived at her office, we were shown into an appointment room and, a few minutes later, Dr. Curry walked in carrying a large manila envelope. She opened the envelope and mounted some transparencies on vertical glass panels and then turned the backlights on to highlight the x-rays.

"Mrs. Carp, the x-rays show that the cancer has spread to your liver."

"Poop," Ruth said. " I have tried so hard to be positive and to think that I could be cured."

"I know, I know," said Dr. Curry. She was close to tears and her voice wavered. "You've always been so upbeat and happy. I hate this part of my job. I am so powerless sometimes. What can I do for you?"

Ruth sat there clutching my hand hard. "Dr. Curry, you have always been honest with me. Tell me, how much time do I have?"

Dr. Curry started to speak, but her voice cracked. She stopped trying to talk, shook her head a few times, dabbed at her eyes with a Kleenex, and then started over. "Six months, Ruth."

Ruth and I both gasped. Her hand clutched my arm harder than it had before.

I moaned to myself, "Why, Goddammit? Why? What has Ruth ever done to deserve this? Why are we being deprived of the ten or twenty years that we deserve?"

Ruth just sat there. I started to weep. Dr. Curry said, "When I was first called in, and I reviewed the medical records, I was guarded about the outcome. You had inflammatory cancer, an especially virulent type. I did not tell you my opinion because you needed to hold on to your hopes. Miracles have happened in the past, and doctors are not always right.

"In your case, I consulted with all of my colleagues hoping that we could come up with a treatment that would stop the cancer from spreading.

"We just don't know enough yet." Dr. Curry's voice shook as she stopped speaking.

I tried, but I couldn't stop the tears from streaming down my face. The news had devastated me. For Ruth's sake, I had to make some attempt to control myself. I wiped my tears and breathed deeply three or four times. I pulled air into my lungs until there was no room for any more, and then slowly exhaled it. I tried to keep my voice strong. "Dr. Curry, Ruth and I want to go back to Carmel, in California. We had such a good time there, before we were married." I stopped. I couldn't go on without breaking down.

Dr. Curry understood immediately. She said, "Jay, you and Ruth make your plans. I can give her medicines so that she will have no pain. If both of you want to go to Carmel, go."

Ruth said quietly, "Dr. Curry, what is next?"

"Ruth, we can start some chemo treatments to try to shrink the cancer. But your veins have taken enough abuse with the needles from the chemo and the blood work. I would suggest that we install a port, a permanent opening we implant in your body to run the chemo treatments through. That way we avoid sticking needles into your veins again."

I don't recall any more of the discussions between Dr. Curry and Ruth. I was crushed and I kept wondering what must Ruth be feeling? She had asked for my strength and I owed it to her for all the joy she had brought me. I had to keep myself together for her sake.

*** 

We left the doctor's office and walked to the car holding hands. We walked slowly neither of us saying a word. As we got to the car, Ruth said, "It just isn't fair. I thought sure that I would beat the cancer. I just get to the time in my life when everything is going well, and I know what happiness is, and then I have to give it up. Shit." She stopped for a second and looked at me. "Oh Honey, I'm so sorry. You got yourself a really bad deal."

I was angry, not with Ruth, but with the entire world. My voice was loud as I replied, "Ruth, I have no idea of what you are talking about. I'm the luckiest man on the face of this fucked up planet. I have you and everything else is bullshit, so don't give me a hard time."

We stood facing each other and both of had tears in our eyes. She smiled, stroked my cheek, and said, "Honey, for goodness sake lower your voice. I only wish that you had called me after we broke up. We could have had all those wasted years together. I love you.

"Now lets try to keep this damn thing on an even keel. When we get home, I will call my girls and talk to them. I still want to go to the lake for our Fourth of July picnic."

She squeezed my hand. "Honey, now you are not only going to have to be strong for me, you are going to have to help my daughters. They will need you in the future as much as I need you now. Until you came back into my life, they had never known a father. They will look to you for help. You will be here for all of us, won't you?"

Ruth kissed me on the cheek, ran her hands over my shoulders, and smiled. I returned her smile as best I could, and nodded my head yes. When I shut the car motor off in our driveway, Ruth sat still for a few seconds and then said, "Jiggety Jog." She turned to look at me and, pointing her finger, continued, "You haven't said your part in over a week. Have you forgotten the words?"

"Jiggety Jig, see I did not forget."

"OK, then, don't overlook them again."

With that, Ruth got out of the car, entered the house, and went into the bathroom. I heard no noise, no water running, no toilet flushing, nothing but silence. I began to get frightened, and I passed by the closed door several times hoping to hear something. As I was getting ready to tap on the door, it opened, and Ruth came out. I could not tell whether or not she had been crying.

She came up to me, kissed me, put her cheek against mine, and said, "Quit being such a worry wart." We stood there hugging each other, wishing our life together would never end.

After a while, Ruth stood back, looked at me, and sighed, "Honey, I am going into the bedroom to call my girls. I will tell them what the doctor told us. Since our picnic is just five days away, I am not going to encourage them to come over now. I will see them then. To tell you the truth, I don't feel too well. I am a little unsteady and nauseous. "After the picnic, you and I will talk about going to Carmel. I really do want to go. But right now, let me concentrate on the picnic and Julie's visit."

My voice would have betrayed my feelings, so I said nothing and pulled Ruth close to me. She hugged me, disengaged herself, and went into the bedroom.

I called my girls that same evening and they took the news very hard. Ruth did not talk to them as she had gone to bed early. The remaining days before the picnic did not go well.

Ruth ate very little and she was sick to her stomach after every meal. Once or twice she went into the bathroom and threw up. I decided that I had to find out how she felt, so I asked. She answered me honestly. She assured me that she was in no pain and that, as long as she could hang in, she was going to the picnic. I wanted to call Dr. Curry, or to take Ruth to the emergency room, but she absolutely refused. She was not about to do anything that might interfere with her picnic.

I didn't press her. Ruth and I both knew that this would be the last picnic she would ever attend. I couldn't, and wouldn't, refuse her. Instead, I swallowed my emotions, shut up, and tried to help.

We would sit for hours doing a crossword puzzle or just talk. Sometimes the black hole of death would recede, but it never did disappear. It was there, ahead of us, looming on our horizon.

Ruth kept saying, "Oh Honey, I am so sorry that you got such a lousy deal. You should have never come to Ann Arbor."

The first few times she said that, I tried to

protest, but that only made her angry. She felt that she was letting me down. I stopped trying to tell her that she was wrong. Although Ruth heard what I said, she did not believe what I said. She felt that I was being cheated, but I knew that her death was cheating both of us.

Because I did not want to upset Ruth, I did not argue. However, I was bound and determined to convince her that I had not been cheated. I decided to let her know how I felt by writing her a letter. At least she could not disagree until after she had read what I had written.

It was easy to find time to collect my thoughts. Ruth wasn't getting up as early as she had in the past. She would remain in bed much longer because of her nausea. I used the time to sort through my feelings so I could tell her exactly how I felt. I mulled over what I was going to write from the time that Edward and Joan had left to go back to New York until the evening of July third. The night before our picnic, I got out a yellow pad of paper, sat down at my desk in the cellar, and wrote Ruth a letter telling her what was in my heart.

Friday was the Fourth of July. While Ruth was in the shower, I straightened out the bedclothes and put the folded note on her pillow. Then I went to the back room, sat down, and pretended to read the newspaper.

After a while Ruth came out of the bathroom and went into the bedroom. I held the newspaper but I was not reading it, I was listening for the normal sounds of Ruth getting dressed, the opening and closing of bureau drawers, or the unzipping of garment bags. I heard only silence, and it seemed to last a long time. Suddenly, Ruth appeared in front of me in her bathrobe and carrying my letter. She may have been crying.

"Honey, thank you for my letter. I love you so very much, Jay Carp."

"Damn it Ruth, quit thanking me." I was brusque because I didn't want to give way to my emotions. Courage and dignity deserve to be answered with courage and dignity. "I am the one who should be thanking you. I just wanted you to know that I did not get a shitty deal and I do not want to hear any more about it."

Ruth smiled, "Well, may I at least thank you for making the bed?"

"You certainly can, and you are more than welcome."

Saturday, the weather was perfect. The sky was clear, the heat was bearable and the humidity was low. The weather was going to be ideal for our picnic. Ruth got up a little later than usual and she was sick to her stomach. She didn't eat much and seemed content to just sit in her easy chair with her eyes closed. Christie and Tracy each called early to find out how their mother was feeling and if she would still be able to go to the lake. Ruth took the calls and assured both of them that she was doing well and that she would be at the picnic. As the time to go got closer, Ruth began to revive and become a little livelier.

We didn't take much with us. In the past, we took food, a big cooler with drinks, fruit, and Ruth's cole slaw, beach paraphernalia, and something to read. This time all we took were two folding chairs, some water, and a beach bag holding sun tan lotion, grapes and our wallets. When I loaded the car, I checked the beach bag to make sure we had everything and I was surprised to see that Ruth had slipped my letter into an inside pocket. She kept the bag by her chair the entire time we were at the lake.

To get to Lake Murray, you have to drive on a private road that winds up a hill to the parking lot for the lake. Just off the public road, the owners have a checkpoint to make sure that only members and guests get to the lake. The owners greeted Ruth enthusiastically. She had been a member for years and, when she hadn't shown up this summer, they had asked Christie and Tracy about her, so they knew that she had cancer. They allowed traffic to build up while they chatted, but they finally had to wave us through because of the backup. Their cheerful greeting made Ruth feel good. As we pulled away, she told me how glad she was to see them again.

We drove up the hill that overlooked the lake and parked at the top. Ruth's daughters had been watching for us, and by the time I stopped our car, Steve, Tracy's husband, and Ruth's two grandsons had run up the hill and were waiting to help Ruth as it was a very steep slope. Ruth protested about all the attention, but I think, secretly, she was pleased. She was weak enough to need the help but stubborn enough not to admit it. When her grandsons, who both stood over six feet four inches tall, each took one of her arms, she laughed and said that anyone watching would think she was drunk. Steve and I carried the chairs and the few other things that we brought with us.

At the edge of the lake, I set up our chairs just within the shade of a big tree, and, once Ruth was seated, her daughters and granddaughters swarmed around her. The little girls were anxious to sit on her lap or to get her attention by grabbing her arm. Christie and Tracy kept reminding their daughters, aged nine and ten, to be gentle with their grandmother. Ruth kept staunchly defending the girls and told her daughters to mind their own damn business.

And so the day passed. It was a day of happiness framed with a fringe of sorrow. Her daughters knew this would be the last picnic ever for the woman who had birthed and raised them. They laughed while reminiscing about their childhood, and, occasionally, they would lapse into a small silence. Ruth had steeled herself for this day, and she acted as if everything was normal. She laughed, asked questions and gave advice without end. She had seized the day and was enjoying it.

When Christie's husband, Richard, finished barbecuing chicken, hamburgers, and hot dogs, we began to eat. Ruth ate more than she had eaten at any time since returning from Russia. She was ravenous devouring deviled eggs, potato salad, chicken, hamburger, and cole slaw; she couldn't get enough to eat. At first, I encouraged her, but soon I became concerned that she would eat too much and get sick. My fears proved to be unnecessary as, eventually, she stopped eating and sat there, relaxed and happy.

Late in the afternoon, Ruth leaned over to me and whispered that she was ready to leave. She told everyone goodbye, and encouraged them to stay as long as they were having a good time. Her grandsons and son-in-laws helped her back up the hill. As she and I were driving to the exit, she said, "That was really nice. I wanted it to be good for them as well as good for me since that will be our last picnic together. Honey, do you think they had a good time?"

I replied, "Ladybug, I am sure they had a good time. Christie and Tracy both told me they were delighted that you were able come."

Ruth patted my knee and then spoke so quietly that I had to strain to hear her, "Honey, I feel so tired and now we have Julie arriving tomorrow. Do you think that she'll be disappointed if I don't do much cooking or entertaining? I really want to, but I don't think that I am up to it."

How does a husband reassure his dying wife that her welfare is more important than making sure the family is entertained? All I could do was reply, "Ruth, Honey, Julie and Michael understand. Don't be concerned; we will manage. You need to take care of yourself."

When we got home, Ruth sat around in her chair for a while, and then she excused herself and got ready for bed. This day had taken a lot out of her and she was not feeling well.

\*\*\*

Sunday was the day that Ruth began to withdraw from life and from me. She stayed in bed not trying to get up except to go to the bathroom. When she woke up in the morning she apologized and said that she did not know if she would be able to visit very much with my daughter and her family. I told her not to worry about it and that I would entertain them. Ruth suggested that I take them sightseeing, especially since Julie had been born at University Hospital in Ann Arbor.

During the day Ruth became less and less communicative. She was quiet, her belly was swollen, and she did not speak unless I spoke to her. When I asked, she told me that she did not feel any pain but that she was a bit nauseous.

In mid afternoon, Julie, Michael and their five-year old daughter arrived. They had driven from North Carolina to attend a wedding in Indiana and they had made a detour on their way back to stop and visit us. It had been planned from the beginning as a very short stay. After spending two or three nights with us they would be leaving to head back to North Carolina. Julie was upset when she saw Ruth even though I had told Julie over the phone that Ruth was dying.

The physical change in Ruth's appearance shocked and disturbed Julie. Ruth had been a vibrant attractive woman when she and Julie had first met. Now, she was a quiet, passive invalid. Julie could not contain her feelings. She saw the angel of death hovering over Ruth and

Julie was unprepared for the sight.

After they unpacked we talked about Ruth and the inevitability of what was going to happen. I fed them, told them to make themselves at home, and then I went to be with Ruth. She held out her hand for me when I entered the bedroom and I took it and sat on the edge of the bed beside her. "Honey, I am sorry that I didn't get out of bed to say 'hello', but I don't feel too well. I hope you told that to Julie and Michael and Grace."

I squeezed her hand a little. "Ladybug, you are one large pain in the ass. Of course Julie understands. She told me to tell you that she loves you, and that she apologizes for whatever she thought or said before she met you."

Ruth smiled. "That was nice of her," she said.

"Well," I replied, " I guess she is a lot like me in that it took her one hell of a long time, but she did get it right. How are you doing?"

"Oh, not too badly."

I thought that she was fibbing for my sake. I changed the subject. "Would you care for something to eat?"

"No thank you Honey, I don't feel like eating anything." She lay there with her eyes closed, not moving at all. I was getting alarmed.

"Ruth, you have been lying in bed all day

without eating anything. You say that you are not having any pain, and I believe you, but I think you ought to let me take you to the emergency room. I think you need to see your doctor."

Ruth just lay there for a while. She had been determined to go to the reunion and the picnic and to see her brother and my daughter. She had done all these things but it had been at a price. Now, she was worn down, not feeling well, and completely drained. She held onto my hand and squeezed it. She whispered, "Honey, why should I go to St. Joseph's? I don't have any pain and there is nothing that they can do for me. It would just mean more work for Dr. Curry, and I would feel foolish."

Foolish? My thoughts arced inside my brain like lightning striking a tree. "Here is my wife, dying, doing the best she can, and being considerate of everyone else. Is this her reward? Is this justice?" I didn't dare linger on those thoughts.

I took several deep breaths and hoped that I sounded normal. "Honey, you shouldn't be the one to judge foolishness. You haven't eaten, you are not feeling well, and you have cancer. Call Dr. Curry and let her decide what to do. I am not a doctor, I know nothing about medicine, but I am sure she will tell you to haul your ass over to the hospital."

Ruth agreed that this would be a reasonable course of action. When she finally reached Dr. Curry, she told Ruth to get to the hospital quickly.

I helped Ruth into the car and drove her to the hospital. She was promptly admitted and they began doing blood tests. When we had talked to Dr. Curry she mentioned the possibility of putting the port in Ruth's neck while she was in the hospital. They gave Ruth a sedative so that she would sleep through the night. I kissed her and left. I had to call all of my daughters.

That night I did not sleep well. I missed having Ruth lying beside me and my thoughts kept me from sleeping most of the night. I woke up early Monday morning feeling logy and with a splitting headache. I quickly showered, told Julie and Michael I would see them later, and left the house because I wanted to have morning coffee with Ruth.

She was awake, feeling better, and anxious to see me. We held hands and she asked about Julie and her family. After some small talk she said she had a story to tell me. One of her nurses was the wife of a doctor, Dr. Berman, for whom Ruth had once worked. He had died several years ago, and his wife, who was a registered nurse, had gone back to work.

We were continually interrupted by a flurry of medical activities. It began as one or two individual tests and, as the results were processed, the necessity of finding more information became apparent. A technician would come in to Ruth's room and say, "We have to have this sample to confirm what we think." Or, "This will tell us about your cell count." The statement was always very narrow, and covered the purpose of the particular test, but it didn't give us any real idea of what was happening. Throughout the day, the tests continued. Most were conducted in her room but a few involved her going on a stretcher to a laboratory.

When she returned to her room after one test in the afternoon, Ruth told me that she felt tired and wanted to sleep. She asked me to go and visit with Julie and come back in the early evening. I kissed her and left so she could get some rest.

I took Julie, Michael, and Grace on a sightseeing tour of Ann Arbor and the University of Michigan. When I took them inside the Michigan football stadium neither could believe the size of the empty bowl and, after I told them that it was going to be enlarged almost ten percent, they were sure that I was kidding them. Michael just kept shaking his head; he couldn't get over what 100,000 empty seats looked like.

Upon my return to Ruth's room, I found

her visiting with several of her friends and three or four flower bouquets on her bedside stand. No one like Ruth can live for almost forty years in a city without leaving many heartprints, all as individual as fingerprints. Ruth's friends, acquaintances, bowling buddies, and co-workers called or came to the hospital. Ruth was glad to see and hear from all of them but the constant flow of visitors meant that we had no time alone. The only good thing about all of the activity was that we were both occupied and distracted from the question of what was happening inside her body.

We found out the next day, Tuesday. Dr. Curry came into Ruth's room and said, "Ruth, Jay, there is no easy way to say this. The tests show that Ruth's cancer is spreading. The spread is so rapid that there is no way to stop it. Putting a port in is not going to help. There is nothing more that can be done."

Ruth lay in bed. I sat in a chair holding her hand. She did not flinch her only movement was to squeeze my hand. I think she realized it before Dr. Curry had said a word. I couldn't help myself, tears rolled down my cheeks.

Dr. Curry explained that they would keep Ruth in the hospital for one or two more days to stabilize the chemical imbalance of her body. That would make her more comfortable and help her feel better. Then, they would discharge her because there were no other medical procedures that would help.

As I sat in stunned silence, Dr. Curry and Ruth were talking. I think Ruth was asking her some questions. I don't know how Ruth managed. I sat there completely overwhelmed. I was like a rock in the rain. I couldn't move. I couldn't protect myself.

When Dr. Curry left, Ruth first squeezed my hand and then she yanked my arm to get my attention. "Honey, yesterday, I never finished telling you about seeing Dr. Berman's wife. She's a nurse on this unit and she went back to work after he died. I hadn't seen her in a few years. Anyhow, I asked her if she ever thought about her husband, and she said 'I think of him every day of my life.'

"Oh Honey, I am so concerned about you."

Agony has to be when your wife is dying and she says she is worried about you. Nothing had ever come close to this stabbing in my heart. I was hopelessly being yanked down a path of pain. I kept silently repeating over and over again, "Ruth is dying. Ruth is dying. Ruth is dying. Ruth is dying."

\*\*\*

Wednesday I stayed with Ruth as much as I could. Early Thursday morning Julie and Michael left to return to North Carolina. When Julie said goodbye she began to cry. She said, "Dad, I am so sorry. I made such a terrible mistake about Ruth. I love her. Do you think she will ever forgive me?" Julie broke down and sobbed uncontrollably.

I held her and said, "Julie, when I showed Ruth the letter you wrote me in California she was hurt and angry. She thought about it for a while and got over her anger. She didn't agree with you, she felt that you had judged her unfairly.

"But, she also said that, since you had lost your mother the way that Virginia died, she couldn't blame you for being protective towards me. All Ruth asked was that you judge her on her own merits. And, over the years, you have. There is nothing to forgive because Ruth has always understood your feelings."

Nothing that I could do or say consoled Julie. She knew she would never see Ruth again. As she drove away from our house she was still crying. I stood in the driveway a long time, staring in the direction they left, overwhelmed with sorrow.

\*\*\*

Later on in the morning, the process of bringing Ruth home from the hospital began. It was complicated because she was scheduled for a few more tests and then she had a meeting to determine the type of medical care she would choose to select after leaving the hospital. She could continue using medicare and our own insurance, or she could accept care from hospice. After listening carefully and asking a lot of questions, Ruth decided to use hospice. We talked with the social director, and she said that tomorrow, a hospice nurse would come to our house to meet with us. In the meantime, some supplies would be sent over to our house later today. It was not until early in the afternoon that we left the hospital. I carried Ruth's bag to the car. On a hunch, I pulled the handles of the bag open and there was the letter that I had written her.

As we pulled into the driveway, Ruth put her hand on my knee and said, "Jiggety jog."

I stopped the car, stared out of the windshield a few seconds, and replied, "Jiggety jig." Ruth squeezed my hand as hard as she could.

"Well, at least I'm home," she said. She sat there a moment, and then she sighed. Ruth patted my leg three or four times, and then said, "Oh Jay Honey, I feel so badly for you."

I wanted to scream, but I didn't. I said as

softly as I could, "Ladybug, please stop saying that."

She smiled at me and replied, "OK, honey. Let's go in the house, I'm feeling tired." Ruth went in and got ready for bed. I could tell that she was not feeling well.

Shortly after we got home, Christie and Tracy came over to visit. They had just returned from a quick trip to New York to pick up Tracy's daughter, Alicia, who had gone back with Joan and Edward to stay with them a few days. Christie and Tracy had driven to New York, picked up Alicia, and drove straight back to Michigan. When they got home they were anxious to see their mother, so they came right over with flowers and little gifts for Ruth. They chatted away, but after a while, seeing that their mother was tiring, they decided to leave. I walked with them to their car. Christie said to me, "Jay, my mommy looks so yellow. I don't ever remember her looking like this before. Is it the cancer that is doing that?"

I put my arms around her shoulder, and replied, "Yes, Christie it is. The cancer has spread to her liver and some of her other organs."

Christie and Tracy were very upset. Christie asked me, "Do you think that we ought to come over and stay with her yet?"

I answered as honestly as I could, "Not yet,

Christie. The time isn't far off, but not right now. I think it would make Ruth mad if she thought that everyone was babying her. I'll let you know when the time comes. It won't be long."

The three of us hugged and cried before they left.

Later on that day, hospice sent over a lot of supplies including oxygen bottles, bandages and a shower chair.

That night Ruth got up several times to go to the bathroom. She was slow to get out of bed, unsteady on her feet, and, when she got inside the bathroom she stayed a long time. When she returned to bed after the third trip, I asked her if she needed help. She absolutely would not hear of it. She said, "I sure as hell don't need anybody giving me assistance when I pee."

She was wrong. Early Friday morning, Ruth went into the bathroom and closed the door. She stayed in the bathroom even longer than she had the on her previous trips. I got up, got dressed, and began pacing around the house, listening for any sound. I would stop near the bathroom door, listen, and worry about Ruth needing help. Then, I would walk away, and, a few minutes later, I would return and listen again. I couldn't tell whether or not Ruth was having problems.

Finally, I heard her say, in a tiny voice,

"Jay, I think I need some help."

I went in and found Ruth, swaying back and forth by the sink. Her nightgown was raised, and her panties were partially pulled down her legs. She had shit herself trying to get to the toilet.

"I am sorry Honey, I can't pull my panties down."

I said quietly, "Oh Ruth darling, don't be sorry. You should have called me earlier. Here, let me help you." I got her panties off and started to clean her up. She was swaying slowly and not saying a word. Knowing how embarrassed she must feel, I kept talking. I am not even sure that what I said made sense. I just wanted to make sure she realized that I was not offended. I got her clean enough to put on another nightgown and get her back to bed.

I did not even attempt to touch the bathroom. I would need help to clean up and to keep an eye on Ruth. I called Christie, and she came as soon as she could. We comforted Ruth, and, when Tracy arrived, the girls got the bathroom cleaned. When they were finished and came into the bedroom to visit Ruth I went down to the cellar and wept.

I thought, "Goddamn it, isn't it bad enough to take her life. Why is it necessary to strip her of her dignity? Why does she have to be mortified? What has she done to deserve such humiliation?" My thoughts were bleak and bitter. I went back upstairs only because I thought that Ruth might need me.

Later that morning, I got a call from hospice and we set up a time for their nurse to come to the house. When I told Ruth the time that the hospice nurse was coming, she said that she wanted to take a shower and clean up before she arrived. Christie and Tracy both wanted to help her, but she refused. The girls placed the shower chair that hospice had delivered inside the tub and Ruth did allow them to help her step over the edge and into the tub. But, then she shut the shower curtain on them. She handed her nightgown out, turned the water on, and took her shower by herself.

When she had finished, she announced to the girls that she wanted to weigh herself. The scales that she insisted on using were in the basement. Ordinarily, she did not like using the basement scales but they read a few pounds lighter than the upstairs scales near the tub; and that was probably why Ruth selected those scales. She needed help going down the cellar stairs and Christie and Tracy had difficulty in getting Ruth over to the scales.

The cellar scales were hard to use. They were electronic and needed to be calibrated before they would weigh anyone. Neither Christie nor Tracy were familiar with the calibration procedure and they would have had problems even if Ruth had been steady on her feet.

They had been in the cellar quite a while when the girls called me and asked for help. They didn't know why they couldn't get the scales to work and Ruth was angry that she couldn't weigh herself. After I showed Christie and Tracy what to do, the three of us were able to get the scales calibrated and Ruth weighed. However, Ruth would not let any of us look at the numbers that the scale registered while she was stranding on it.

Christie told me later that, after the first attempt to weigh her mother had failed, Ruth had said, "Oh fuck." And she had gotten madder after each subsequent failure. In an attempt to calm Ruth down, Christie told her that it really wasn't too important to get weighed. "It doesn't have to be done now," Christie had said.

Ruth looked at her and said, "You have time Christie, but I don't." Christie felt awful. After Christie told me this story, she broke down and cried. I tried to comfort her by telling her that Ruth had not meant that as a rebuke but only as a fact. Nothing I said comforted Christie.

Later that Friday, the nurse from hospice arrived and Ruth talked with her and answered all of her questions. The nurse set up an elaborate medicinal schedule for the weekend, she gave me a list of instructions along with a phone number for us to call if we had any questions. Then she was gone and we were on our own. Christie and Tracy stayed beside their mother as much as they could; they knew that they were going to lose her soon and they couldn't bear to let her out of their sight. They wanted to be with her every possible second while she was still breathing. The thought of not having their mother in their lives terrified them. They did not leave the house from that Friday evening until the following Monday when Ruth died.

\*\*\*

After the hospice nurse left, the girls helped Ruth into bed and we started the complicated schedule of medications that the nurse had written out for us. Some medicines were to be given alone, other medicines were to be given in combinations, and some of the combinations required changing the medicine dosage. In addition, there were medicines to be given if Ruth had pain or if she did not respond to the other medications. What bothered us so much was that all of the medicines were to be administered on the basis of the patient's responses. We could not determine Ruth's responses. She just lay in bed with her eyes closed, not talking and not answering our questions. The three of us were confused, uncomfortable and apprehensive.

It was shortly after Ruth was put to bed that she became almost comatose. She responded to our questions and comments only a few times. We were anxious about whether we were administering the medications correctly and we couldn't tell if she were in pain, or if she were thirsty, or what her needs were. We hovered around Ruth, trying to determine if she was even aware of us.

That evening, the girls slept in the bedroom in the cellar and I slept with Ruth. I patted her cheek, kissed her hand, and told her that I loved her. She did not respond in any way. I began to smell the fumes and feel the heat of the fires of Hell.

Saturday we were frenzied as we tried to comply with the schedules for administering the medicines. Many times that day, I called the number the hospice nurse had given us and talked with the duty nurses. They were patient and thorough, but I never felt reassured when I finished talking with them. I don't believe the nurses understood the gravity of Ruth's condition and our confusion didn't help them. The one thing that I didn't do, and have wished many times since that I had done, was to ask them to come over and assist us. It never entered my mind and they never volunteered.

We were frightened because Ruth was not responding to our conversations or our touches. We tried to be cheerful when we were in the bedroom, but we cried in all the other rooms. Each of us knew we were losing Ruth. I cried because love is so very beautiful when you have it but so very painful when it is stolen from you.

Christie called Robin, in Atlanta, and told her that their mother was slipping rapidly, more rapidly than we had expected or been led to believe. Christie told Robin to leave for Ypsilanti immediately. It is a fifteen-hour drive to get here from Atlanta. Robin and said she would leave at once.

As bad as Saturday was for us, Sunday was worse. Ruth lay in bed hardly moving. Her skin was yellow and now we could see that her lips were dry. We would moisten them and try to keep her comfortable, all the while not knowing if we were of any help. Not only were we fighting our fears and sorrows we were also fighting the panic of helplessness. Since Friday evening, when we started administering Ruth's medications, we were not sure we were doing the job correctly. We needed Ruth's responses to help us determine the amounts of the doses, and she was unconscious. We were in a frenzy to keep her comfortable, with no pain, but we did not know exactly what to do.

Beginning early Sunday morning, Christie, Tracy, and I took turns calling the hospice nurse. Each time she responded to our questions and made suggestions for us to follow. We tried to follow their advice, but with Ruth being unresponsive, we couldn't tell what we were doing. And never once did I have the common sense to ask them to come over.

Robin arrived during the afternoon, and, after taking one look at her mother, she broke down in tears. It was a shock for Robin to see her mother lying in bed, comatose, yellow skinned, with her belly swollen by the cancer that was killing her. Robin never got the chance to talk with her mother or even say goodbye. By that evening, Ruth's breathing started to become erratic. We talked to hospice and we clumsily followed every direction they gave us. None of us slept that evening.

Monday morning, the nurse who had seen Ruth on Friday returned. She was taken aback by the change in Ruth's condition. She told us that Ruth's death was imminent, and she immediately called her office and cancelled her other appointments. She would stay with us until the end. Close to noontime, Ruth passed away.

After she died, I went into the bedroom

to say my final goodbye to the person who had been my wife, my companion, and my friend. On the bed lay the bloated and yellowed corpse of a sixty-eight year old woman. That was not what I saw. I saw a tall, blond girl so alive, so vivacious, and so beautiful that she had taken my breath and stolen my heart. That will always be my picture of Ruth.

When the undertaker arrived, Christie took off Ruth's engagement and wedding rings and gave them to me. Sometime later, Dr. Curry signed the death certificate that stated Ruth died of breast cancer. As Ruth requested, she was cremated.

And now, for me, all that is left is a paraphrase of Philippians, IV. 7.

"The pain of God, which passeth all understanding."

\*\*\*

*July 4, 1997*

*Dearest Ruth,*

*Ever since I returned to Michigan, and found you again, you have questioned my explanation for even passing through this area.*

*"You really came to visit my Mother?" You always asked. Sometimes you would grin, some-*

*times you would shake your head, sometimes you would slap my forearm lightly; but you would always have an air of disbelief.*

*As naïve and as dumb as it now seems, it is the truth. I had actually intended to see your mother, visit with you, and then go on to my house in Santa Maria. When I arrived in Ypsilanti I was a middle-aged man who had married, raised a family, buried a wife, and retired. I was alive, but I assumed that I had used up my quota of joy and happiness. I had thought that old age was to be an arid landscape with no great swings of feelings or emotions.*

*What I discovered in Ypsilanti was something I never expected. I found you. And what made finding you so deliciously sweet was that I had not only found you once I was lucky enough to have found you twice.*

*The first time was when we were both young and I was green and callow. I was lost in my awe of you. Your beauty, your intelligence, your sense of humor scorched my tongue and addled my thoughts. I loved you then, but I was not mature, and so, I lost you.*

*The second time we met was as equals, and the fire that had been quenched for over forty years ignited for both of us. You rekindled my love for you and my zest for life.*

*We became partners, and what a happy part-*

*nership it has been. We were man and woman, husband and wife, and best of friends. We were so close physically, mentally, and spiritually, that our hearts beat almost as one.*

*Lately, you have been telling me that I got a bad bargain in marrying you. My reply to you Ruth, is "No, and Hell no." Our time together has been bliss. You have made me the happiest man in the world, not just once, but twice.*

*I lost you once and it took a long time for the pain to fade. Now, I am going to lose you again. This time the pain may fade, but it will not disappear. The joy of knowing you, loving you, being with you, and having you as my wife will never leave me. I wish we had gone on for a million days; but I am so grateful for the days that you did give me. I have been blessed with the gift of Ruth.*

*I will carry your love and your spirit with me for the rest of my days. They will guide me and help me in my times of need. I will try to be good and do only the things that you would want me to do.*

*My darling Ruth, as we always say when you and I touch our glasses and make our toast,*

*"Klunk, I love you."*

## *Epilogue*

It has been almost twelve years since Ruth died.

No human being can suffer the death of a mate without being diminished in heart and soul and for years I was bitter and angry.

However, as my ache lessened I had to face the fact that Ruth and I were no longer husband and wife. Our love and our life together would be remembered as memories.

I also knew that Ruth would absolutely not want me wallowing in self-pity. She would be adamant that I live my life fully and that I do the best I can until my own time came.

To that end, for mankind I ask for peace, for my friends and family I hope for happiness, for myself I search for love.

## About the Author

After earning degrees from the University of Michigan in both LSA and School of Engineering, Jay Carp joined General Telephone ad electronics (GTE), where he remained for over thirty years working in military electronics. His career took him around the world, including to Thule, Greenland to work on the Ballistic Missile Early Warning System (BMEWS). He was also part of the teams to develop a radar system for use in Viet Nam to locate enemy mortar and artillery shells.

For twenty years, Mr. Carp worked entirely on Inter Continental Ballistic Missile (ICBM) systems. When the Minuteman missile was first deployed at the Air Base in Grand Forks, North Dakotas, he was working directly with the Strategic Air Command (SAC). His experiences gave him an understanding of the Air Force operational problems over and above any technical consideration and full familiarity with Minuteman, MX, Peacekeeper and Rail Garrison missile systems.

During the years Mr. Carp worked on

ICBM's, he was a field engineer, test supervisor, troubleshooter, project engineer and project manager. His last field assignment prior to retirement was a GTE Site Manager at Vandenberg Air Base in California.

Jay Carp resides in Milan, Michigan where he remains a loving Dad to his six daughters and their children — three daughters by his first wife Virginia and three acquired by marriage to Ruth.

Jay Carp is the author of *COLD WAR CONFESSIONS - Inside Our Classified Defense Programs* a National Best Book of 2007 Finalist Award Winner.

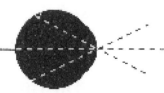

# N.A.V.H. Seal of Approval

*Celebrating 50 Years*

**National Association for Visually Handicapped (N.A.V.H.) is a nonprofit health organization. Our mission is to ensure that impaired vision does not lead to impaired life. Our services help the "hard of seeing" overcome the psychological and physical barriers to maintaining independence.**

**New York National Headquarters**
**22 West 21st Street    6th floor**
**New York, New York 10010**

**212-889-3141**
**888-205-5951**

**Fax: 212-727-2931**
**navh@navh.org**

# *Jay Carp*

# The Gift of Ruth